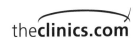
theclinics.com

CARDIOLOGY CLINICS

The Athlete's Heart: On the Border
Between Physiology and Pathology

GUEST EDITOR
Antonio Pelliccia, MD

CONSULTING EDITOR
Michael H. Crawford, MD

August 2007 • Volume 25 • Number 3

SAUNDERS

An Imprint of Elsevier, Inc.
PHILADELPHIA   LONDON   TORONTO   MONTREAL   SYDNEY   TOKYO

W.B. SAUNDERS COMPANY
A Division of Elsevier Inc.

Elsevier Inc. • 1600 John F. Kennedy Blvd., Suite 1800 • Philadelphia, Pennsylvania 19103-2899

http://www.theclinics.com

CARDIOLOGY CLINICS   Volume 25, Number 3
August 2007   ISSN 0733-8651
Editor: Barbara Cohen-Kligerman   ISBN-13: 978-1-4160-5042-1
                                                            ISBN-10: 1-4160-5042-6

Reprints. For copies of 100 or more, of articles in this publication, please contact the Commercial Reprints Department, Elsevier Inc., 360 Park Avenue South, New York, New York 10010-1710. Tel. (212) 633-3813 Fax: (212) 462-1935 email: reprints@elsevier.com.

The ideas and opinions expressed in *Cardiology Clinics* do not necessarily reflect those of the Publisher. The Publisher does not assume any responsibility for any injury and/or damage to persons or property arising out of or related to any use of the material contained in this periodical. The reader is advised to check the appropriate medical literature and the product information currently provided by the manufacturer of each drug to be administered to verify the dosage, the method and duration of administration, or contraindications. It is the responsibility of the treating physician or other health care professional, relying on independent experience and knowledge of the patient, to determine drug dosages and the best treatment for the patient. Mention of any product in this issue should not be construed as endorsement by the contributors, editors, or the Publisher of the product or manufacturers' claims.

Cardiology Clinics (ISSN 0733-8651) is published quarterly by Elsevier Inc., 360 Park Avenue South, New York, NY 10010-1710. Months of issue are February, May, August, and November. Business and editorial Offices: 1600 John F. Kennedy Blvd., Suite 1800, Philadelphia, PA 19103-2899. Customer Service Office: 6277 Sea Harbor Drive, Orlando, FL 32887-4800. Periodicals postage paid at New York, NY, and additional mailing offices. Subscription prices are $226.00 per year for US individuals, $344.00 per year for US institutions, $113.00 per year for US students and residents, $276.00 per year for Canadian individuals, $418.00 per year for Canadian institutions, $301.00 per year for international individuals, $418.00 per year for international institutions and $150.00 per year for Canadian and foreign students/residents. To receive student/resident rate, orders must be accompanied by name of affiliated institution, data of term, and the *signature* of program/residency coordinator on institution letterhead. Orders will be billed at individual rate until proof of status is received. Foreign air speed delivery is included in all *Clinics* subscription prices. All prices are subject to change without notice. POSTMASTER: Send address changes to *Cardiology Clinics*, Elsevier Periodicals Customer Service, 6277 Sea Harbor Drive, Orlando, FL 32887-4800. **Customer Service: 1-800-654-2452 (US). From outside of the US, call 1-407-345-1000.**

Cardiology Clinics is also published in Spanish by McGraw-Hill Interamericana Editores S. A., P.O. Box 5-237, 06500, Mexico D. F., Mexico; in Portuguese by Reichmann and Alfonso Editores Rio de Janeiro, Brazil; and in Greek by Dimitrios P. Lagos, 8 Pondon Street, GR115-28 Ilissia, Greece.

Cardiology Clinics is covered in *Index Medicus, Excerpta Medica, The Cumulative Index to Nursing and Allied Health Literature* (INAHL).

Printed in the United States of America.

CONSULTING EDITOR

MICHAEL H. CRAWFORD, MD, Professor of Medicine, University of California San Francisco; Lucie Stern Chair in Cardiology, and Interim Chief of Cardiology, University of California San Francisco Medical Center, San Francisco, California

GUEST EDITOR

ANTONIO PELLICCIA, MD, Institute of Sport Medicine and Science, Italian National Olympic Committee, Rome, Italy

CONTRIBUTORS

ALLEN E. ATCHLEY, Jr, MD, Fellow, Division of Cardiovascular Medicine, Duke University Medical Center, Durham, North Carolina

AARON L. BAGGISH, MD, Fellow in Cardiovascular Medicine, Department of Cardiology, Massachusetts General Hospital, Boston, Massachusetts

CRISTINA BASSO, MD, PhD, Associate Professor of Cardiovascular Pathology, Department of Medical-Diagnostic Sciences and Special Therapies, University of Padova Medical School, Padua, Italy

ALESSANDRO BIFFI, MD, Institute of Sports Medicine and Science, Italian National Olympic Committee, Rome, Italy

ELISA CARTURAN, BSc, PhD, Research Fellow, Department of Medical-Diagnostic Sciences and Special Therapies, University of Padova Medical School, Padua, Italy

DOMENICO CORRADO, MD, PhD, Associate Professor of Cardiology, Department of Cardio-Thoracic and Vascular Sciences, University of Padova Medical School, Padua, Italy

F.M. DI PAOLO, MD, Institute of Sport Medicine and Science, Italian National Olympic Committee, Rome, Italy

PAMELA S. DOUGLAS, MD, Ursula Geller Professor of Research in Cardiovascular Diseases, Duke University Medical Center, Durham, North Carolina

N.A. MARK ESTES III, MD, Professor of Medicine, The New England Cardiac Arrhythmia Center, Division of Cardiology, Tufts-New England Medical Center, Boston, Massachusetts

ROBERT H. FAGARD, MD, PhD, Professor of Medicine, Faculty of Medicine, Hypertension and Cardiovascular Rehabilitation Unit, Department of Cardiovascular Diseases, University of Leuven, Leuven, Belgium

HEIN HEIDBÜCHEL, MD, PhD, Cardiology - Electrophysiology, University Hospital Gasthuisberg, University of Leuven, Leuven, Belgium

MARK S. LINK, MD, Associate Professor of Medicine, The New England Cardiac Arrhythmia Center, Division of Cardiology, Tufts-New England Medical Center, Boston, Massachusetts

BARRY J. MARON, MD, Director, Hypertrophic Cardiomyopathy Center, Minneapolis Heart Institute Foundation, Minneapolis, Minnesota; and Professor of Medicine, Tufts University School of Medicine, Boston, Massachusetts

PIERANTONIO MICHIELI, MD, PhD, Center for Sports Medicine and Physical Activity Unit, Social Health Department, Padova, Italy

ANTONIO PELLICCIA, MD, Institute of Sport Medicine and Science, Italian National Olympic Committee, Rome, Italy

MAURIZIO SCHIAVON, MD, Center for Sports Medicine and Physical Activity Unit, Social Health Department, Padova, Italy

GAETANO THIENE, MD, FRCP Hon, Professor of Cardiovascular Pathology, Department of Medical-Diagnostic Sciences and Special Therapies, University of Padova Medical School, Padua, Italy

PAUL D. THOMPSON, MD, Division Chief, Department of Cardiology, Henry Low Heart Center, Hartford Hospital, Hartford, Connecticut

CONTENTS

> The athlete's heart is a constellation of cardiac morphologic changes, including increased left ventricular volume, increased left ventricular mass, increased left atrial volume, and right ventricular structural changes as a physiologic response to exercise training. These structural changes fall within the normal reference ranges of appropriately matched control subjects for most trained individuals; however, there are significant numbers of athletes who have "abnormal" measurements. The ability to distinguish between physiologic changes associated with the athlete's heart and structural abnormalities that may represent underlying cardiac disease is of paramount importance. Structural heart disease significantly increases risk for morbidity, mortality, and sudden death, especially during exercise or physical stress. This article reviews the morphologic changes associated with the athlete's heart.

> Long-term athletic training is associated with changes in cardiac morphology, commonly described as "athlete's heart." Although numerous studies have investigated the effects of training on cardiac dimensions, most are limited to male Caucasian athletes, and few data are available regarding the effect of long-term exercise training on the woman's heart. This article reviews the athlete's heart in relation to gender and race.

> The Italian screening protocol has adequate sensitivity and specificity for detection of potentially dangerous cardiovascular diseases, and substantially reduces mortality of

young competitive athletes, mostly by preventing sudden cardiac death from cardiomyopathy. The results of the Italian preparticipation evaluation program have significant implications worldwide: this article addresses the efficacy and feasibility of preparticipation screening, essentially based on 12-lead ECG, as has been in practice in Italy for 25 years.

Cardiovascular disease is the most frequent cause of death in young athletes, and hypertrophic cardiomyopathy (HCM) is the single most common condition responsible for these tragedies. Detection of diseases such as HCM can be achieved in general athlete populations through preparticipation screening, and most effectively if testing with electrocardiography or echocardiography is incorporated into the process. Criteria for disqualification and eligibility, based on identified cardiovascular abnormalities, are available in consensus panel guidelines for both United States and European athletes. Removal from intense training and competition is recommended for athletes with HCM, some of whom may ultimately be judged to be at unacceptably high risk for sudden death and eligible for prophylactic defibrillator implantation.

This article examines the role of arrhythmogenic right ventricular cardiomyopathy/dysplasia in causing sudden death in young competitive athletes and suggests a prevention strategy based on identification of affected athletes at preparticipation screening. Systematic cardiovascular screening (including 12-lead ECG) of all subjects embarking on sports activity has the potential to identify those athletes at risk and to reduce mortality.

This article focuses on uncommon heart diseases associated with an increased risk for sudden death during exercise, namely, myocarditis and dilated cardiomyopathy.

The augmentation of myocardial function that accompanies vigorous exercise is dependent upon adequate coronary artery blood flow reserve. Coronary artery pathology may limit coronary blood flow and produce myocardial ischemia. The clinician charged with the care of athletes must have a high index of suspicion for underlying coronary artery pathology when faced with an individual with suggestive symptoms. This article discusses diseases of the coronary circulation relevant to athletes.

FORTHCOMING ISSUES

RECENT ISSUES

ELSEVIER
SAUNDERS

Cardiol Clin 25 (2007) ix

CARDIOLOGY
CLINICS

Foreword

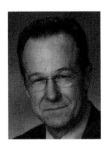

Michael H. Crawford, MD
Consulting Editor

Consultative cardiologists frequently encounter patients in whom a component of their "abnormal findings" may be due to the effects of athletic training. I recently saw a young man with a large right ventricle and what looked like an atrial septal defect on transthoracic echocardiography. His history revealed intense athletic training and transesophageal echo showed a patent foramen ovale. Clearly, his right heart enlargement was due to his exercise training and not the patent foramen. He did not need this foramen closed.

The topic of the athlete's heart has been covered in two earlier issues of the *Cardiology Clinics* that were guest edited by Dr. Barry Maron. Recently, there has been considerable data on this topic emanating from Italy, which has the most organized sports medicine program of any country in the world. Thus, I was delighted when Dr. Antonio Pelliccia, who has generated much of this data, agreed to guest edit this issue on the athlete's heart. He has assembled experts from all over the world to cover topics in three basic areas: the physiology of the athlete's heart, clinical issues, and how to manage these individuals. There is considerable practical information concerning how to screen athletes for cardiovascular disease and how to manage problems such as syncope, tachyarrhythmias, and hypertension in athletes. Also, there are separate articles on the three important cardiomyopathies that can lead to sudden death in athletes: hypertrophic, arrhythmogenic right ventricular, and dilated. In addition, the issue of ischemic heart disease is discussed, since athleticism at older ages is becoming more common. Finally, there is a discussion about the use of internal cardioverter defibrillators in athletes, which has become an important legal issue.

I am confident that you will enjoy this world-class issue on a complex problem that is frequently seen today because of increased exercise and sports participation all over the world.

Michael H. Crawford, MD
Division of Cardiology
Department of Medicine
University of California
San Francisco Medical Center
505 Parnassus Avenue, Box 0124
San Francisco, CA 94143-0124, USA

E-mail address: crawfordm@medicine.ucsf.edu

CARDIOLOGY
CLINICS

Cardiol Clin 25 (2007) xi–xv

Preface

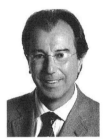

Antonio Pelliccia, MD
Guest Editor

The athlete's heart is one of the most intriguing and stimulating topics in clinical cardiovascular medicine. The effects of chronic exercise on the heart were initially investigated in animal models at the end of twentieth century, and scientists recognized that wild animals have an enlarged and hypertrophied heart in comparison to domesticated animals. For instance, the heart weight of the hare is double that of a rabbit of similar age and weight [1].

The first description in humans of cardiac changes associated with exercise training and sport competition date as far back as 1899, when S. E. Henshen, Professor of Medicine at the University of Uppsala, published the report *A Study in Sports Medicine; Skiing and Competitive Skiing*, in which he stated that "skiing causes an enlargement of the heart and this enlarged heart can perform more work than a normal heart. There is, therefore, a physiologic enlargement of the heart due to athletic activity" (ie, the "*athlete's heart*") [2]. This accurate definition is impressive when we consider that Henshen assessed heart size in cross-country skiers uniquely by carefully performed chest percussion!

Subsequently, Scandinavian scientists F. Rohrer and A. Kahlstorf introduced radiologic techniques to assess heart volume in athletes [3]. Cardiac volume was routinely assessed with radiography in athletes participating in the 1928 Olympic Games in Amsterdam, and the concept was raised that cardiac size differed in athletes according to the type of sporting discipline in which they participated, with athletes engaged in endurance sports (such as long distance running, cycling, or swimming) showing the most enlarged hearts [4,5]. Assessment of cardiac volume with radiography was largely used by Reindell and subsequently by Hollman, who confirmed the original observations of Deutsch and Herxheimer and added the concept that enlarged cardiac size was associated with improved physical performance, in that athletes who showed the greatest increase in radiographic heart volume also showed the highest aerobic capacity, as expressed by maximum oxygen uptake [6,7].

However, the concept that sport activity was responsible, per se, for a purely physiologic cardiac remodeling was largely controversial within the scientific community. Several scientists expressed concern regarding the intrinsic nature and long-term clinical consequences of morphologic cardiac changes observed in athletes, and referred to this issue as *athlete's heart syndrome*. Dietlen, for instance, refused to believe that dilatation of the heart was a physiologic adaptation and postulated that participation in strenuous sport activity would, over time, result in a deterioration of cardiac function and predisposition to heart failure [8]. As recently as 1972, the concept that cardiac dimensional increase in athletes "is likely the consequence of a rheumatic, syphilitic or congenital heart disease" was expressed in a major textbook of cardiology edited by Friedberg [9]. Moreover, cardiovascular morbidity was believed to be greater in trained athletes, in spite of the lack of epidemiologic studies supporting this view.

Substantial contributions to the clinical issues surrounding the athlete's heart were made in Italy in the 1930s, when the first manual dedicated to the evaluation of athletes, *Controllo medico dello sport* (*Medical Evaluation in Sport*), was published by Ugo Cassinis [10] and subsequently in the 1960s when Antonio Venerando performed serial radiologic and electrocardiographic studies on athletes participating in the 1960 Olympic Games in Rome [11]. Based on the privileged observatory of the Institute of Sport Medicine, Venerando and colleagues (Fig. 1) made several intriguing observations. A variety of cardiac radiographic silhouettes were described in trained athletes, in selected cases mimicking those found in patients with valvular or congenital heart disease, and raising the

question of differential diagnosis [12]. The electrocardiographic studies of Olympic athletes showed a large proportion of sinus bradycardia, increased R/S wave voltages in precordial leads, and delayed AV conduction, which were considered benign expressions of the athlete's heart. Indeed, certain alterations were also associated with the athlete's heart, such as the second-degree AV block or the diffusely inverted T waves in precordial/standard leads (Fig. 2) [13]. Such observations unavoidably raised new scientific debate and received enormous scientific attention at the International Conference of Sports Cardiology, held in Rome in 1978.

Echocardiography, introduced in clinical cardiovascular medicine at end of the 1970s, gave great impulse to investigation of the morphologic and functional features of the athlete's heart, with Rost being one of the pioneer cardiologists who investigated the echocardiographic dimensional changes in athletes according to age and type of sport [14]. In 1975, Morganroth and colleagues [15] published the first comparative echocardiographic

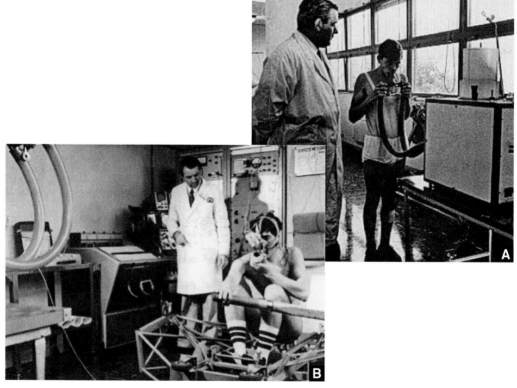

Fig. 1. (*A*) Professor Antonio Venerando and (*B*) Professor Antonio Dal Monte at work at the Institute of Sports Medicine in 1966.

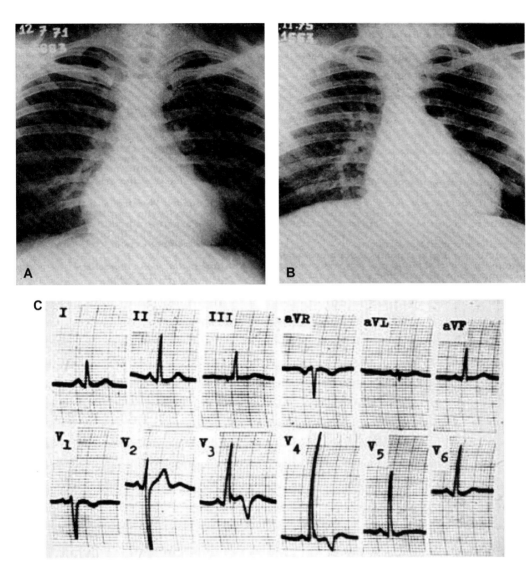

Fig. 2. Chest radiographs from (*A*) a 27-year-old male professional cyclist showing a symmetrically enlarged cardiac silhouette and (*B*) a 24-year-old male elite water polo player showing an enlarged cardiac silhouette suggestive of distinctly enlarged left ventricle dimensions. (*C*) A 12-lead echocardiogram recorded in a 32-year-old male athlete participating at the 1960 Olympic Games in Rome showing diffusely markedly abnormal repolarization pattern in association with increased R/S wave voltages in precordial leads V2–V5.

study of cardiac dimensions in athletes engaged in endurance-type and strength-type sports in the *Annals of Internal Medicine*. This investigation pioneered a large series of studies assessing the mechanisms, upper limits, and clinical correlates of cardiac remodeling in trained athletes according to type of sport, sex, and age. In this context, a study describing the characteristics and upper limits of left ventricular hypertrophy in the largest athlete cohort was published in 1991 in the *New*

England Journal of Medicine [16]. The largest investigation describing the athlete's heart in women appeared in 1995 in *JAMA: the Journal of the American Medical Association* [18] and, subsequently, a report on the upper limits and clinical correlates of left ventricular dilatation was published in 1999 in the *Annals of Internal Medicine* [17].

A new impetus for understanding the clinical issues surrounding the athlete's heart was provided by reports describing adverse cardiac events (ie, sudden cardiac death occurring in apparently healthy, young competitive athletes). In the 1970s, Jokl and McClellan [19] initially described the ominous occurrence of cardiac death during exercise. This controversial problem of contemporary cardiovascular medicine received greatest visibility, however, in 1980, when *Circulation* published Maron's momentous paper, in which the most common diseases responsible for such deaths were reported [20].

In subsequent years, this issue has attracted great attention, and several surveys have extensively described the spectrum of cardiac pathologic conditions associated with sudden death in athletes [21,22]. Thus, timely recognition of the structural cardiac abnormalities responsible for such catastrophes, together with criteria for the differential diagnosis of athlete's heart have become the most critical issue, with relevant medical, legal, economic, and ethical implications.

Prevention of unexpected, sudden death in young athletes is presently one of the most widely debated clinical issues in cardiovascular medicine applied to athletes (*sport cardiology*) and has prompted new debate regarding the feasibility, efficacy, and practicability of preparticipation cardiovascular screening. To address this problem, the American Heart Association and the European Society of Cardiology have recently published position statements for physicians in the United States and Europe, respectively [23,24]. Moreover, the appropriate management of athletes with known cardiovascular disease represents a challenging problem in current clinical practice and has been approached by expert panels appointed by the American Heart Association and European Society of Cardiology, respectively. As a result, consensus documents were recently published, intended to offer scientific advice and legal defense to clinicians who are required to evaluate athletes with known cardiovascular abnormalities [25,26].

This issue of the *Cardiology Clinics* is designed to offer a comprehensive overview of the most debated and controversial clinical issues surrounding the athlete's heart and to provide updated information to clinical cardiologists, general practitioners, and sport scientists on how to correctly differentiate the physiologic cardiac remodeling induced by competitive sport from structural cardiac diseases, as well as the criteria to appropriately manage athletes with recognized cardiovascular abnormalities.

Antonio Pelliccia, MD
Italian National Olympic Committee
Institute of Sport Medicine and Science
Largo P. Gabrielli 1
Rome 00197, Italy

E-mail address: antonio.pelliccia@coni.it

References

[1] Scheuer J, Tipton CM. Cardiovascular adaptations to physical training. Annu Rev Physiol 1977;39: 221–51.

[2] Henschen S. Skilanglauf und Skiwettlauf. Eine medizinische Sportstudie. Mitt Med Klin Upsala (Jena) 1899;2:15–8.

[3] Rohrer F. Volumenbestimmung an Korperhohlen und Organen auf orthodiagraphischem wege. Fortschr Rontgenstr 1916;24:285–9.

[4] Deutsch F, Kauf E. Herz und Sport. Bern: Wien; 1924.

[5] Buytendijk FJJ, Snapper I. Ergebnisse sportarztlichen Untersuchungen bei den IX Olympischen Spielen in Amsterdam 1928. Berlin: Springer; 1929.

[6] Reindell H, Klepzig H, Steim H, et al. Herz-Kreislaufkrankheiten und Sport. Munich; Barth: 1960.

[7] Hollman W. Der arbeits und trainingseinfluss auf Kreislauf und Atmung. Darmstadt (Germany): Dr. Steinkopff; 1959.

[8] Dietlen H, Moritz F. Über das Verhalten des herzen nach langandauerndem und anstrengendem Rad fahren. Munch Med Wochenschr 1908;55:489–93.

[9] Friedberg C. Erkrankungen des Herzens. 2 Aufl. Stuttgart (Germany): Thieme; 1972.

[10] Cassinis U. Controllo Medico dello Sport. Rome (Italy): Enzo Pinci Ed; 1934.

[11] Venerando A, Rulli V. Frequency, morphology and meaning of the electrocardiographic anomalies found in Olympic marathon runners. J Sports Med 1964;3:135–41.

[12] Rossi F, Todaro A, Venerando A. Pulmonary circulation in endurance athletes. J Sports Med 1997;17: 269–73.

[13] Zeppilli P, Fenici R, Sassara M, et al. Wenckebach second-degree A-V block in top-ranking athletes: an old problem revisited. Am Heart J 1980;100: 281–94.

[14] Rost R, Schneider K, Stegmann N. Vergleichende echokardiographische Untersuchengen am Herzen del Leistungsportlers und des Nichttrainierten. Med Welt 1972;23:1088–93.

[15] Morganroth J, Maron BJ, Henry WL, et al. Comparative left ventricular dimensions in trained athletes. Ann Intern Med 1975;82:521–4.

[16] Pelliccia A, Maron BJ, Spataro A, et al. The upper limit of physiologic cardiac hypertrophy in highly trained elite athletes. N Engl J Med 1991;324: 295–301.

[17] Pelliccia A, Culasso F, Di Paolo F, et al. Physiologic left ventricular cavity dilatation in elite athletes. Ann Intern Med 1999;130:23–31.

[18] Pelliccia A, Maron BJ, Culasso F, et al. Athlete's heart in women: echocardiographic characterization of highly trained elite female athletes. JAMA 1996; 276:211–5.

[19] Jokl E, McClellan JT. Exercise and Cardiac Death. JAMA 1970;213:1489–91.

[20] Maron BJ, Roberts WC, McAllister HA, et al. Sudden death in young athletes. Circulation 1980;62: 218–29.

[21] Maron BJ, Shirani J, Poliac LC, et al. Sudden death in young competitive athletes: clinical, demographic and pathologic profiles. JAMA 1996;276:199–204.

[22] Maron BJ. Sudden death in young athletes. N Engl J Med 2003;349:1064–75.

[23] Maron BJ, Thompson PD, Ackerman MJ, et al. Recommendations and considerations related to preparticipation screening for cardiovascular abnormalities in competitive athletes: 2007 update.

A scientific statement from the American Heart Association council on nutrition, physical activity and metabolism. Endorsed by the American College of Cardiology Foundation. Circulation [published on line, March 12, 2007; DOI: 10.1161/CirculationAHA.107.181423].

[24] Corrado D, Pelliccia A, Bjornstad HH, et al. Cardiovascular pre-participation screening of young competitive athletes for prevention of sudden death: proposal for a common European protocol. Consensus Statement of the Study Group of Sport Cardiology of the Working Group of Cardiac Rehabilitation and Exercise Physiology and the Working Group of Myocardial and Pericardial Diseases of the European Society of Cardiology. Eur Heart J 2005;26:516–24.

[25] Maron BJ, Zipes DP. 36th Bethesda Conference. Eligibility recommendations for competitive athletes with cardiovascular abnormalities. J Am Coll Cardiol 2005;45:1312–75.

[26] Pelliccia A, Fagard R, Bjørnstad HH, et al. A European Society of Cardiology consensus document: recommendations for competitive sports participation in athletes with cardiovascular disease. Eur Heart J 2005;26:1422–45.

ELSEVIER
SAUNDERS

CARDIOLOGY
CLINICS

Cardiol Clin 25 (2007) 371–382

Left Ventricular Hypertrophy in Athletes: Morphologic Features and Clinical Correlates

Allen E. Atchley, Jr, MD[a], Pamela S. Douglas, MD[b],*

[a]Division of Cardiovascular Medicine, Duke University Medical Center, Box 31037, Durham, NC 27710, USA
[b]Division of Cardiovascular Medicine, Duke University Medical Center, Box 3850, Durham, NC 27710, USA

Cardiac enlargement and hypertrophy in response to prolonged exercise training have been described for more than 100 years. Physicians at the turn of the century, such as Henschen and Osler [1,2], made these observations based primarily on careful history and physical examination. The development and technologic refinement of echocardiography throughout the 1970s and 1980s provided the methodology for a detailed evaluation of the morphologic and functional milieu of the heart in trained athletes. A constellation of findings known as the athlete's heart was described, including increased end diastolic dimensions of the right and left ventricle, left ventricular hypertrophy, increased left ventricular mass, and increased volume of the left atrium with preserved systolic and diastolic function. Although these structural changes commonly represent a physiologic process in young and otherwise healthy athletes, they can also represent pathologic cardiovascular disease. The athlete's heart has been a subject of much study over the past several decades as the ability to differentiate a pathologic process from an otherwise benign physiologic process is of critical importance to the clinician and patient.

Morphologic changes of the athlete's heart represent physiologic adaptation to increase the efficiency of the heart and vascular system, in part in response to increases in volume and peripheral resistance with intense athletic training. The crux of such an adaptation is the ability to increase oxygen delivery by way of increased cardiac output. This can be expressed by the Frank-Starling Law, which explains the heart's ability to increase contractile force and stroke volume in response to increased volume and mechanical stretch, and by the Fick principle, in which oxygen consumption is expressed as a function of cardiac output times the difference between oxygen content of the arterial and mixed venous blood ($VO_2 = CO \times AV\ O_2$ difference). Of the structural changes previously listed, all contribute to increased efficiency of cardiovascular function through the Starling mechanism, with the exception of left ventricular hypertrophy (LVH). Increased left ventricular thickness, however, reduces myocardial wall tension that occurs with increased chamber size at a given pressure, as expressed by the law of Laplace (in which wall tension = pressure × radius/thickness) [3].

Changes in cardiac morphology vary significantly with the type of exercise training (ie, isotonic versus isometric), sex, and body size. Although these differences may be statistically significant, most findings associated with the athlete's heart fall within the normal reference ranges for appropriately matched control subjects. In trained individuals who have morphologic features that are clearly abnormal, or even in an intermediate "gray zone," the possibility of a pathologic process must be considered. The differential diagnosis for such individuals includes structural heart disease, such as dilated cardiomyopathy, hypertrophic cardiomyopathy, arrhythmogenic right ventricular cardiomyopathy (ARVC), and myocarditis. Preserved systolic and diastolic function and regression of structural abnormalities with deconditioning are consistent with

---

* Corresponding author.
E-mail address: pamela.douglas@duke.edu
(P.S. Douglas).

physiologic adaptation to training. Persistence of pathologic findings warrants cessation of sports activity and further investigation for potential genetic or treatable disease processes that may have a significant impact on morbidity and mortality, especially with respect to arrhythmia and sudden death.

Left ventricle

Increased left ventricular end diastolic dimension in trained athletes has been well documented in numerous studies over the past several decades [4–15]. In 1999, Pelliccia and colleagues [13] studied 1309 elite male and female athletes from 38 different sports and ages ranging from 13 to 59 years. In this study there was a significant degree of variability in the left ventricular diastolic dimension, with a mean of 48 mm (range, 38–66 mm) in women and a mean of 55 mm (range, 43–70 mm) in men. Most of these athletes (55%) had dimensions that fell within the accepted upper limit of normal (<54 mm). Only 14% of the athletes in this study had left ventricular end diastolic dimensions greater than 60 mm, and dilatation greater than this is considered uncommon (Fig. 1) [8,12,13]. In a recent study of 442 highly trained British athletes from 13 different sports by Whyte and colleagues [14] in 2005, only 5.8% of male athletes had an end diastolic dimension greater than 60 mm with an absolute upper limit of 65 mm. None of the 136 female athletes from this study had an end diastolic diameter greater than 60 mm.

Left ventricular wall thickness can also be increased in elite athletes. Pelliccia and colleagues [10] demonstrated that the vast majority, more than 98%, of trained individuals had a left ventricular wall thickness of 12 mm or less.

Although left ventricular mass in trained individuals is also usually within accepted normal limits, hypertrophy has been noted [8,10,12,13]. Douglas and colleagues examined 235 highly trained triathlon participants and found that 32 (16%) had septal wall measurements greater than 1.1 cm and only 2 (<1%) had septal wall thickness exceeding 1.3 cm. In the same group of athletes only 7 (3%) had a posterior wall thickness greater than 1.1 cm, and only 1 had a posterior wall thickness exceeding 1.3 cm [12].

The normal range of left ventricular mass as calculated from echocardiographic measurements for non-athlete control subjects has been well established in studies such as the Framingham Heart Study [16]. Given that cardiac mass is calculated as a function of wall thickness and end diastolic dimension, it stands to reason that increased cardiac mass is a common finding in trained athletes who have increased LV size. In a meta-analysis of 59 studies including more than 1450 athletes, Pluim and colleagues [17] demonstrated a highly significant difference ($P < .001$) in cardiac mass between trained athletes (249 g) when compared with control subjects (174 g). This difference seems to be more pronounced in female athletes, because cardiac mass can vary significantly with respect to height and body surface area. Among 235 triathlon participants studied by Douglas and colleagues [12], 43% of females had an absolute LV mass greater than the accepted upper limits of normal (198 g) and only 17% of males had an absolute LV mass that exceeded accepted upper limits of normal (294 g) (Fig. 2). Like other morphologic changes associated with athlete's heart, LV mass thus usually falls within the accepted normal limits for age- and sex-matched control subjects, and LV hypertrophy, if present, is usually mild

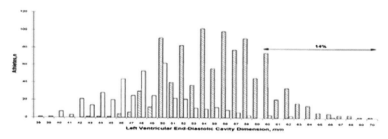

Fig. 1. Distribution plot of left ventricular end diastolic dimension in a group of highly trained male (*hatch*) and female (*white*) athletes. Results demonstrating that approximately 14% of individuals studied have an end diastolic dimension that is markedly enlarged, greater than 60 mm. (*From* Pelliccia A, Culasso F, Di Paolo FM, et al. Physiologic left ventricular cavity dilatation in elite athletes. Ann Intern Med 1999;130:23; with permission.)

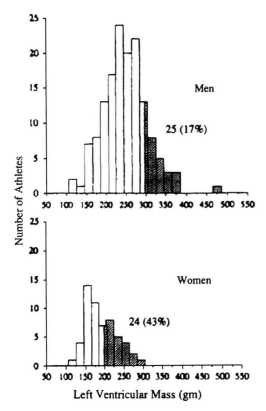

Fig. 2. Distribution plots of un-normalized left ventricular mass for 235 male and female ultra distance triathletes. Athletes who had left ventricular hypertrophy, according to calculated mass >294 g in men and >198 g in women, marked with hatched bars. (*From* Douglas PS, O'Toole ML, Katz SE, et al. Left ventricular hypertrophy in athletes. Am J Cardiol 1997;80:1384; with permission.)

to moderate at worst [4–15]. In addition, concentric and eccentric remodeling is rare. In Douglas and colleagues' study [12], the septal-to-posterior wall thickness ratio was normal (<1.3) in 98% of athletes (Fig. 3). Further analysis for potential eccentric remodeling was performed by calculating a relative wall thickness ratio in which the septal and posterior dimensions are averaged and plotted against cavity radius. A value of less than 0.30, indicating significant eccentric remodeling, was seen in 15 (7%) athletes (Fig. 4). Other determinants of LVH, such as sex, type of exercise, and genetics, are discussed later in this review.

Cardiac MRI is a rapidly growing and evolving technology for evaluating cardiac structure and function that has been used in several studies to evaluate LV morphology in athletes and control subjects (Fig. 5) [18,19]. Data from these studies

are similar to the previously established values by evaluation with echocardiography.

LV systolic function is generally preserved in trained athletes in the face of increased cavity dimension, wall thickness, and mass [4–15]. This serves as an important point of differentiation between potentially pathologic changes with respect to cardiac morphology versus benign physiologic adaptation to exercise training. There have been small studies that demonstrated reduced contractile indices in trained individuals [20,21]. These findings, however, are believed to be because indices used for the noninvasive assessment of LV function can depend on volume load, which may be altered in trained individuals. When load-independent measures of LV function, such as stress shortening relationships, have been studied, no abnormalities in myocardial contractility were observed [22].

LV diastolic function has been well studied in athletes since the introduction of noninvasive modes of evaluation with echocardiography. Impairment of diastolic function has been demonstrated in individuals who have increased LV end diastolic dimension, LVH, or increased LV mass when these changes occur in the setting of other cardiac diseases, such as systemic hypertension, aortic stenosis, coronary ischemia, or other primary myocardial diseases [23–27]. Any or all of these morphologic changes, however, can be observed in trained athletes with no adverse effect on diastolic function [7,28–33]. Instead, several studies evaluating transmitral flow by Doppler echocardiography have shown higher early peak diastolic filling velocity and higher ratios of early-late filling velocities (E/A ratio usually 1.5:1.9) in trained athletes when compared with non-athlete control subjects [28,31–33], suggesting supranormal diastolic function. In another study, Granger and colleagues [29] compared 11 athletes who had LVH and increased cardiac mass (mean, 127 g/m^2) versus 12 control subjects who had substantially lower cardiac mass (mean, 82 g/m^2) and found no difference between the two groups with respect to diastolic filling rate. Preservation of LV diastolic function in the athlete's heart is therefore an important point of distinction from cardiac morphologic changes that may represent an underlying pathologic process.

Left atrium

Left atrial enlargement is another common morphologic finding in the heart of trained

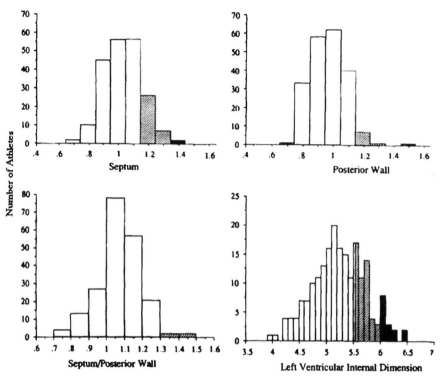

Fig. 3. Distribution plots of septal and posterior wall thickness (*upper left and right panels*) and septum/posterior wall thickness ratio and left ventricular end diastolic dimension (*lower left and right panels*). Normal values are shown in white, abnormal values are hatched, and markedly abnormal values are black. (*From* Douglas PS, O'Toole ML, Katz SE, et al. Left ventricular hypertrophy in athletes. Am J Cardiol 1997;80:1384; with permission.)

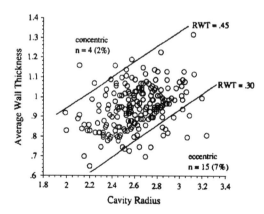

Fig. 4. Scatter plot of average left ventricular wall thickness versus cavity radius. The upper line represents a relative wall thickness (RWT) >0.45, above which concentric remodeling is present, and the lower line represents an RWT of 0.30, below which eccentric remodeling is present. (*From* Douglas PS, O'Toole ML, Katz SE, et al. Left ventricular hypertrophy in athletes. Am J Cardiol 1997;80:1384; with permission.)

athletes [4–15,34–36]. The degree of enlargement is usually mild to moderate and within accepted normal limits when compared with non-athlete control subjects. Increased diameter of the left atrium is found more commonly in athletes who have demonstrable changes in LV morphology and in those individuals active in ultra-endurance sports activities (ie, cycling and marathon running) and is believed to be secondary to increased volume load. In 2005, Pelliccia and colleagues [22] evaluated left atrial dimensions in 1777 athletes from 38 different sports. Left atrial dimensions were 37±4 mm in male athletes (71%) and 32±4 mm in female athletes. Mild to moderate left atrial enlargement (>40 mm) was common, occurring in approximately 20% of athletes, but significant enlargement (>45 mm) was uncommon, occurring in only 2% of those examined (Fig. 6). In the same study the occurrence of atrial fibrillation or supraventricular tachycardia was rare, with an overall incidence of less than 1% [22,35]. Morphologic changes of the left atrium thus seem to be part of

Endurance Athlete   **Untrained Control Subject**

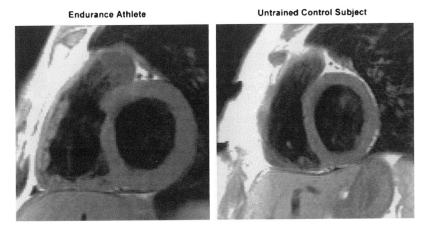

Fig. 5. End diastolic T-1 weighted short axis cardiac MRI images demonstrating the left and right ventricular morphologic changes associated with the athlete's heart (*left*) compared with that of an untrained control subject (*right*). These changes include increased left and right ventricular end diastolic dimension, increased left and right ventricular hypertrophy, and increased left ventricular mass in trained athletes. (*From* Scharhag J, Schneider G, Urhausen A, et al. Athlete's heart: right and left ventricular mass and function in male endurance athletes and untrained individuals determined by magnetic resonance imaging. J Am Coll Cardiol 2002;40(10):1856–63; with permission. Copyright © 2002 American College of Cardiology Foundation.)

the normal physiologic adaptation of the heart and vascular system in response to exercise training.

Right ventricle

The right ventricle of trained athletes has been evaluated in many studies [8,9,37–46]. In general, findings with respect to right ventricular

morphology and function in the athlete's heart include mild to moderate increases in end diastolic volume and wall thickness with preserved contractile function. Adequate assessment of the right ventricle by way of transthoracic echocardiography can be technically challenging because of its irregular shape [42–45]. As previously outlined, cardiac MRI has been used to evaluate LV morphology and mass in trained and untrained

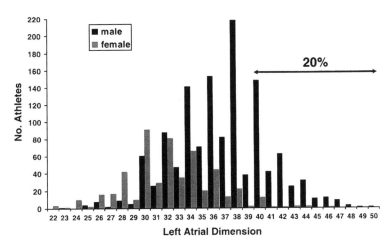

Fig. 6. Distribution plot of left atrial dimension in a group of highly trained male (*dark bar*) and female (*gray bar*) athletes. Approximately 20% of individuals have enlarged left atrial dimension greater than 40 mm, with only 2% showing marked left atrial enlargement greater than 45 mm. (*From* Pelliccia A, Maron BJ, DiPaolo FM, et al. Prevalence and clinical significance of left atrial remodeling in competitive athletes. J Am Coll Cardiol 2005;46:690–6; with permission. Copyright © 2005 American College of Cardiology Foundation.)

individuals, but studies evaluating the right ventricles of athletes are limited. In 2002, Scharhag and colleagues [38] evaluated right ventricular structure and function in 21 trained athletes who had cardiac MRI and compared the findings to untrained control subjects. They found a significant increase in right ventricular end diastolic volume of approximately 25% in trained individuals versus control subjects (mean volumes of 160 mL versus 128 mL, respectively). Right ventricular mass was also increased by approximately 37% in trained athletes versus control subjects (mean gram weight of 77 and 56 g, respectively) (Fig. 5). Overall right ventricular systolic function was comparable in both groups. Mild to moderate structural changes of the right ventricle therefore occur in response to exercise training, including increased end diastolic volume, wall thickness, and mass, all of which should be considered normal physiologic adaptation as part of the athlete's heart complex.

Morphologic changes with different types of exercise training

The type of exercise training is one of the most significant factors in determining the type and extent of morphologic changes in the athlete's heart [5,6,8,11,13,14,17,22,28,34,37]. In general, training that is predominantly isotonic (aerobic) in nature leads to more significant changes in LV cavity dilatation, wall thickness, and mass. This is in contrast to athletic activities in which the training is predominantly isometric (strength) in nature in which there may be only increased wall thickness. These differences are believed to be caused by the increased cardiac output and volume demand in isotonic training versus the increased pressure and afterload associated with isometric training, although for most athletes, training and competition represent a combination of the two forms of exercise. The observation that cardiac morphologic changes varied with respect to the type of exercise training was first noted by Morganroth and colleagues [5] in 1975. This finding has been further demonstrated in several studies, including a study of 947 athletes from 27 different sports by Spirito and colleagues [11], which demonstrated that the most significant increases in LV cavity and wall thickness were observed in sports, such as cycling, rowing, and cross-country skiing, whereas sports such as weight lifting and wrestling induced less significant changes and the effects on wall thickness predominated (Fig. 7).

Body size and sex

Body size and sex are also major determinants on the absolute cardiac morphologic changes associated with the athlete's heart [7,8,10–15,47]. In general, larger male athletes have greater

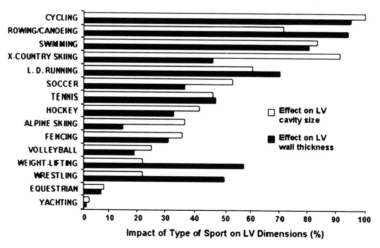

Fig. 7. Graph representing effects of different types of sports training on left ventricular cavity size (*light bar*) and left ventricular wall thickness (*dark bar*). Overall the greatest degree of left ventricular cavity size in wall thickness is associated with ultra-endurance aerobic activities, especially those involving upper extremity exercise. (*From* Maron BJ, Pelliccia A. The heart of trained athletes: cardiac remodeling and the risks of sports, including sudden death. Circulation 2006;114:1633–44. Reproduced from the American Heart Association, Inc.; with permission.)

absolute increases in LV wall thickness, cavity dimension, mass, and left atrial dimension (see Figs. 2, 3, and 6). Like other morphologic changes with the athlete's heart, LV mass per body surface area is significantly enlarged when compared with control subjects but usually falls within the accepted normal values for these measurements (<150 g/m^2 for men and <120 g/m^2 for females). Cardiac changes associated with the athlete's heart are otherwise not routinely scaled with respect to body surface area, although, because extremes of body size are often advantageous, athletes may represent outliers when compared with the population average (eg, jockeys versus basketball players). In a study of 600 female athletes from various different sports activities, trained individuals had significantly increased end diastolic dimension and wall thickness when compared with non-athletic sex-matched control subjects. The same female athletes, however, were found to have significantly smaller cavity dimensions, wall thicknesses, and mass when compared with more than 700 male athletes who were involved in similar sports activities [47]. Although it could be conceived that the differences in cardiac morphology between male and female athletes were primarily caused by differences in body size (body surface area or height), Spirito and colleagues [11] demonstrated that female athletes of similar body size from the same sport had a smaller LV end diastolic dimension and wall thickness than male counterparts.

Genetic determinants

The extent and variability of morphologic changes that occur in the heart of trained athletes is in large part explained by differences in body size, type of sport activity, and gender [13,34]. There is, however, a significant degree of variability among athletes that cannot be explained by these factors alone. Other genetic and environmental factors are believed to have a significant role in the cardiac structural changes in athletes also. In 1997, Montgomery and colleagues [48] evaluated 140 military recruits before and after a 10-week period of strength and endurance training. Overall the group had mild to moderate increases in LV end diastolic dimension, wall thickness, and mass. The group was then evaluated with respect to genotype by different polymorphisms of the angiotensin converting enzyme (ACE) gene. These polymorphisms included deletion (D) or insertion (I) of a marker where its absence (D) was associated with higher circulating and tissue concentrations of ACE. This study demonstrated a significant difference in LV wall thickness and mass between the different genotypes. Overall LV mass in the homozygous II group was increased by 2 g, in the heterozygous ID group by approximately 38 g, and in the homozygous DD group by 42 g after exercise training. Similar findings have been shown with polymorphisms of the angiotensinogen gene also [49,50]. There is much more to be learned about the genotype and resultant phenotypic expression in the athlete's heart, but underlying genetic determinants likely play a large role in the degree to which cardiac structural changes may be observed in addition to body size, sex, and type of exercise training.

Athlete's heart and structural cardiac disease

The ability to distinguish between the adaptations in cardiac morphology associated with exercise training from those related to pathologic heart disease is one of the most critical aspects in evaluating the heart of elite athletes. As previously discussed, the heart of a trained individual usually falls within accepted normal limits, including the following measurements: end diastolic dimension less than 6.0 cm, LV wall thickness less than 1.3 cm, septal–posterior wall thickness ratio less than 1.3, relative wall thickness between 0.30 and 0.45, and LV mass less than 294 g in men and 198 g in women [51]. There can be, however, significant overlap between the upper limits of "normal" in the athlete's heart with other forms of structural cardiac disease. In contrast to the assessment of systolic function, which is often normal in questionable cases, diastolic function can be a powerful discriminator between physiologic and pathologic hypertrophy. The enhanced filling seen in athletes is easily separated from the impaired relaxation and altered filling pattern associated with most forms of myocardial disease or ischemia [7,28–33]. In addition to systolic and diastolic function assessment, other strategies have been used to help differentiate the physiologic changes associated with exercise training from pathologic changes of other structural heart diseases.

Regression of morphologic changes associated with the athlete's heart after cessation of training has been described in several small studies [52–54]. In the largest of these studies, Pelliccia and colleagues [52] evaluated 40 elite athletes who had LV enlargement greater than 6.0 cm or LV wall thickness greater than 1.3 cm with serial echocardiography for an average of 5.6 years after cessation of exercise training. All of these individuals had normalization of LV wall thickness and decreased end diastolic dimension (Fig. 8). Of the 9 athletes (22%) who had persistent end diastolic dimension greater than 6 cm, more than half could be potentially explained by increases in body weight or ongoing recreational exercise activity. There seemed to be no adverse long-term cardiovascular sequelae associated with the morphologic changes of the athlete's heart during the follow-up period.

Cardiac MRI is a rapidly emerging and evolving technology with many applications, some of which include assessment of cardiac structure and

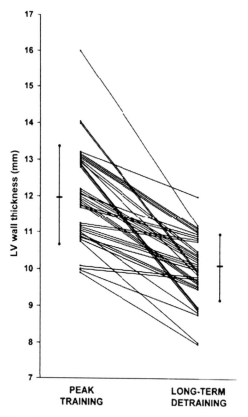

Fig. 8. Regression of left ventricular wall thickness associated with detraining over an average of approximately 5 years. (*From* Pelliccia A, Maron BJ, de Luca R, et al. Remodeling of left ventricular hypertrophy in elite athletes after long-term deconditioning. Circulation 2002;105:944–9. Reproduced from the American Heart Association, Inc.; with permission.)

function. In 2005, Petersen and colleagues [55] examined a total of 120 individuals who had cardiac MRI, including 18 healthy control subjects, 25 athletes who had LVH, and 77 patients who had LVH in the setting of underlying cardiovascular disease (hypertrophic cardiomyopathy, aortic stenosis, or hypertension). In their analysis, a receiver-operating curve was used to define an LV diastolic wall thickness to cavity volume ratio of less than 0.15 mm/m^2/mL as normal. This resulted in an area under the curve of 0.993 and the ability to correctly distinguish morphologic changes of the athlete's heart from those associated with other underlying cardiovascular disease with a sensitivity of 80% and a specificity of 99%. This study could not, however, distinguish between etiologies of LV enlargement among those who had underlying cardiovascular disease. Cardiac MRI therefore could be a useful tool in evaluating individuals who have athlete's heart and in distinguishing the morphologic changes associated with exercise training from those found in other underlying pathologic cardiovascular diseases.

Another more novel way of potentially differentiating morphologic changes of the athlete's heart from structural cardiac disease is serum measurement of N-terminal pro-brain natriuretic peptide (NT-proBNP). NT-proBNP is released from cardiac myocytes in response to increased ventricular wall stress and can lead to significantly elevated serum concentrations in pathologic forms of structural heart disease [52]. In 2004, Scharhag and colleagues [56] evaluated serum concentrations of NT-proBNP in 20 trained endurance athletes and compared those results to 20 otherwise healthy untrained control subjects. The trained individuals had cardiac structural changes suggestive of athlete's heart as determined by evaluation with cardiac MRI. The results revealed that there was no significant difference in the serum concentrations of NT-proBNP between the two groups with a mean concentration of 24.7 pg/mL in athletes versus 28.9 pg/mL in the controls (P = .56). There may be increases in serum BNP on initiation of intense training as was demonstrated by Montgomery and colleagues [48] in their study of British military recruits, but this finding was also in conjunction with a high prevalence of the ACE "D" gene allele and elevated myocardial mass. Although more study is needed, measurement of NT-proBNP serum concentrations in chronically trained athletes may be a useful adjunct in differentiating pathologic from adaptive cardiac morphologic changes.

Clinical correlates

Exercise training conveys an unequivocal mortality benefit over time [53]. There is, however, a significant increase in the risk for sudden death during exercise activity [34,54,57–60]. This risk varies with age, occurring in less than 1 per 100,000 in young individuals and approximately 6 per 100,000 in older individuals [58]. The difference between the two groups is primarily caused by the increasing incidence of coronary artery disease with aging. Although the absolute increase in sudden death associated with exercise is small, owing primarily to the relative infrequency of such events, the relative risk can be increased by approximately 2 to 10 times that of sedentary individuals [58]. Despite the transient increase in mortality associated with exercise, the overwhelming benefit of chronic exercise training is an overall decrease in mortality. In a large meta-analysis of 44 observational studies with cohorts ranging from several hundred to more than 30,000, an inverse linear dose-response relationship between exercise and all-cause mortality was observed. From this study it was further concluded that even mild to moderate amounts of exercise, approximately 1000 kilocalories of energy expenditure per week, could convey a 20% to 30% reduction in mortality [61]. Even though there is a small but significant absolute increase in sudden death associated with exercise training, this risk is believed to be far outweighed by the long-term survival benefit conveyed by chronic physical training. Although there has been debate over the potential clinical implications of the structural changes associated with the athlete's heart, the long-term mortality benefit associated with exercise underscores the high probability that these changes are adaptive and physiologic in nature for most trained individuals.

Most studies of athletes are cross-sectional rather than longitudinal. The long-term effects of a sustained, high level of exercise training in middle aged and older athletes are far less well delineated than those of training for only a few years and in younger individuals. To address this, a recent preliminary report compared 108 marathon runners older than age 50 years (mean age, 57 years) who had no known coronary artery disease against 424 matched sedentary control subjects. The athletic cohort was noted to have significantly reduced risk factor profiles for the presence of coronary disease with decreased BMI (−14%), decreased systolic blood pressure (−10%), decreased LDL (−18%), and increased HDL (42%). Despite the favorable risk factor profile, the marathoners had a significantly greater amount of subclinical coronary atherosclerosis as defined by the prevalence of a cardiac CT coronary artery calcium (CAC) score of greater than 100 (36.2% versus 22.2%; $P < .003$) [60]. This raises an important question about the potential need for screening older athletes for the presence of coronary disease despite their apparent health. These data have only been published in abstract form, however, so that confirmation in another cohort and further study are needed to elucidate the validity and clinical implications of these initial findings.

Nevertheless, these cautionary data support current guideline recommendations for a more careful assessment of the older individual before exercise. These include pre-participation screening in athletic activities for individuals of advanced age using a thorough history and physical examination and a baseline electrocardiogram [62]. Further investigation with a symptom limited maximal exercise ECG stress test is recommended for individuals who have symptoms consistent with underlying coronary artery disease or in asymptomatic men aged 40 to 45 years and older and women aged 50 to 55 years and older with one or more risk factors for the development of coronary artery disease (ie, hypertension, tobacco use, family history, diabetes mellitus, and dyslipidemia).

Summary

The athlete's heart is a physiologic adaptation in response to chronic exercise training that is comprised of morphologic changes, including increased LV volume, increased LV mass and hypertrophy, increased left atrial volume, and right ventricular structural changes. Several factors such as body size, sex, type of exercise (aerobic versus isometric), and even genotype can greatly influence the degree to which these changes may be observed. In general, these structural changes fall within the normal reference ranges of appropriately matched control subjects. There are, however, a small number of trained individuals who have significant cardiac enlargement that could potentially represent pathologic cardiac disease. In these cases the ability to differentiate structural cardiac disease from normal adaptation to training is paramount, with the increased risk for morbidity and mortality associated with underlying cardiovascular disease. Various measures are available to make this important determination, including cessation of training (detraining) with serial examination to evaluate for regression of structural changes, further evaluation of geometric indices and functional parameters with echocardiography or cardiac MRI, and serologic evaluation with NT-proBNP.

The clinical implications of athlete's heart are important, because there is a significant acute and transient increase in the risk for sudden death associated with exercise. The risk in young athletes is largely from structural diseases, such as hypertrophic cardiomyopathy, arrhythmogenic right ventricular cardiomyopathy, and coronary anomalies. In older athletes, the risk is higher than in younger counterparts, with coronary artery disease being the most significant risk factor, for which there are currently no specific screening recommendations other than a thorough history and physical examination. Despite the cardiac morphologic changes and acute risk for sudden death associated with exercise training, there is an unequivocal mortality benefit associated with long-term exercise training and the potential benefits of physical activity far outweigh the risks.

References

[1] Henschen S. Skidlauf und Skidwettlauf. Eine medizinische Sportstudie. Mitt Med Klin Upsala 1899;2:15.
[2] Osler W. The principles and practice of medicine. New York: D. Appleton and Company; 1892.
[3] Puffer JC. Overview of the athletic heart syndrome. In: Thompson PD, editor. Exercise and sports cardiology. New York: McGraw-Hill Companies; 2001. p. 43–70.
[4] Raskoff WJ, Goldman S, Gohn K. The "athletic heart:" prevalence and physiologic significance of left ventricular enlargement in distance numbers. JAMA 1976;236:158–62.
[5] Morganroth J, Maron BJ, Henry WL, et al. Comparative left ventricular dimensions in trained athletes. Ann Intern Med 1975;82:521–4.
[6] Keul J, Dickhuth HH, Simon G, et al. Effect of static and dynamic exercise of heart volume, contractility, and left ventricular dimensions. Circ Res 1981; 48(Suppl I):I162–70.
[7] Douglas PS, O'Toole ML, Hiller WD, et al. Left ventricular structure and function by echocardiography in ultraendurance athletes. Am J Cardiol 1986; 58:805–9.
[8] Maron BJ. Structural features of the athlete heart as defined by echocardiography. J Am Coll Cardiol 1986;7:190–203.
[9] Douglas PS, O'Toole ML, Hiller WD, et al. Different effects of prolonged exercise on the right and left ventricles. J Am Coll Cardiol 1990;15:64–9.
[10] Pelliccia A, Maron BJ, Spataro A, et al. The upper limit of physiologic cardiac hypertrophy in highly trained elite athletes. N Engl J Med 1991;324: 295–301.
[11] Spirito P, Pelliccia A, Proschan MA, et al. Morphology of the "athlete's heart" assessed by echocardiography in 947 elite athletes representing 27 sports. Am J Cardiol 1994;74:802–6.
[12] Douglas PS, O'Toole ML, Katz SE, et al. Left ventricular hypertrophy in athletes. Am J Cardiol 1997;80:1384–8.
[13] Pelliccia A, Culasso F, Di Paolo FM, et al. Physiologic left ventricular cavity dilatation in elite athletes. Ann Intern Med 1999;130:23–31.
[14] Whyte GP, George K, et al. The upper limit of physiological cardiac hypertrophy in elite male and female athletes: the British experience. Eur J Appl Physiol 2004;92:592–7.
[15] Ghorayeb N, Batlouni M, Pinto IM, et al. Left ventricular hypertrophy in athletes: adaptive physiologic response of the heart. Arq Bras Cardiol 2005;85(3):191–7.
[16] Levy D, Savage DD, Garrison RJ, et al. Echocardiographic criteria for left ventricular hypertrophy: the Framingham Heart Study. Am J Cardiol 1987;59: 956–60.
[17] Pluim BM, Zwinderman AH, van der Laarse A, et al. The athlete's heart: a meta-analysis of cardiac structure and function. Circulation 1999;100:336–44.
[18] Milliken MC, Stray-Gundersen J, Peshock RM, et al. Left ventricular mass as determined by magnetic resonance imaging in male endurance athletes. Am J Cardiol 1988;62:301–5.
[19] Lorenz CH, Walker ES, Morgan VL, et al. Normal human right and left ventricular mass, systolic function, and gender differences by cine magnetic resonance imaging. J Cardiovasc Magn Reson 1999;1:7–21.
[20] Gilbert CA, Nutter DO, Felner JM, et al. Echocardiographic study of cardiac dimensions and function in the endurance-trained athlete. Am J Cardiol 1977; 40:528–33.
[21] Nishimura T, Yamada Y, Kawai C. Echocardiographic evaluation of long-term effects of exercise on left ventricular hypertrophy and function in professional bicyclists. Circulation 1980;61:832–40.
[22] Colan SD, Sanders SP, Borow KM. Physiologic hypertrophy: effects on left ventricular systolic mechanics in athletes. J Am Coll Cardiol 1987;9: 776–83.
[23] Hanrath P, Mathey PG, Siegert R, et al. Left ventricular relaxation and filling pattern in different forms of left ventricular hypertrophy: an echocardiographic study. Am J Cardiol 1980;45:15–23.

[24] Maron BJ, Spirito P, Green KJ, et al. Noninvasive assessment of left ventricular diastolic function by pulsed Doppler echocardiography in patients with hypertrophic cardiomyopathy. J Am Coll Cardiol 1987;10:733–42.

[25] Eichorn P, Grimm J, Koch R, et al. Left ventricular relaxation in patients with left ventricular hypertrophy secondary to aortic valve disease. Circulation 1982;65:1395–404.

[26] Inouye I, Massie B, Loge D, et al. Abnormal left ventricular filling: an early finding in mild to moderate systemic hypertension. Am J Cardiol 1984;53: 120–6.

[27] Fifer MA, Borow KM, Colan SD, et al. Early diastolic ventricular function in children and adults with aortic stenosis. J Am Coll Cardiol 1985;5: 1147–54.

[28] Colan SD, Sanders SP, MacPherson D, et al. Left ventricular diastolic function in elite athletes with physiologic cardiac hypertrophy. J Am Coll Cardiol 1985;6:545–9.

[29] Granger CB, Karimeddini MK, Smith VE, et al. Rapid ventricular filling in left ventricular hypertrophy. J Am Coll Cardiol 1985;5:862–8.

[30] Matsuda M, Sugishita Y, Koseki S, et al. Effect of exercise on left ventricular diastolic filling in athletes and nonathletes. J Appl Physiol 1983;55:323–8.

[31] Vanoverschelde JJ, Essamari B, Vanbutsele R, et al. Contribution of left ventricular diastolic function to exercise capacity in normal subjects. J Appl Physiol 1993;74:2225–33.

[32] Nixon JV, Wright AR, Porter TR, et al. Effects of exercise on left ventricular diastolic performance in trained athletes. Am J Cardiol 1991;68:945–9.

[33] Forman DE, Manning WJ, Hauser R, et al. Enhanced left ventricular diastolic filling associated with long-term endurance training. J Gerontol 1992;47(2):56–8.

[34] Maron BJ, Pelliccia A. The heart of trained athletes: cardiac remodeling and the risks of sports, including sudden death. Circulation 2006;114:1633–44.

[35] Pelliccia A, Maron BJ, DiPaolo FM, et al. Prevalence and clinical significance of left atrial remodeling in competitive athletes. J Am Coll Cardiol 2005;46:690–6.

[36] Mont L, Sambola A, Brugada J, et al. Long-lasting sport practice and lone atrial fibrillation. Eur Heart J 2002;23:477–82.

[37] Fagard R. Athlete's heart. Heart 2003;89:1455–61.

[38] Scharhag J, Schneider G, Urhausen A, et al. Athlete's heart right and left ventricular mass and function in male endurance athletes and untrained individuals determined by magnetic resonance imaging. J Am Coll Cardiol 2002;40(10):1856–63.

[39] Ector J, Ganame J, van der Merwe N, et al. Reduced right ventricular ejection fraction in endurance athletes presenting with ventricular arrhythmias: a quantitative angiographic assessment. Eur Heart J 2007;28:345–53.

[40] Sahn DJ, DeMaria A, Kisslo J, et al. Recommendations regarding quantitation in M-mode echocardiography: results of a survey of echocardiographic measurements. Circulation 1978;58:1072–83.

[41] Mumford M, Prakash R. Electrocardiographic and echocardiographic characteristics of long distance runners. Comparison of left ventricular function with age- and sex-matched controls. Am J Sports Med 1981;9:23–8.

[42] Kasikcioglu E. A difficult puzzle: right ventricular remodeling in athletes. Int J Cardiol 2005;103(1):114.

[43] Henriksen E, Landelius J, Wesslen L, et al. Echocardiographic right and left ventricular measurements in male elite endurance athletes. Eur Heart J 1996; 17:1121–8.

[44] Kasikcioglu E, Oflaz H, Akhan E, et al. Right ventricular Tei index in athletes. Echocardiography 2004;21:373.

[45] D'Andrea A, Caso P, Sarubbi B, et al. Right ventricular adaptation to different training protocols in top-level athletes. Echocardiography 2003;20: 329–36.

[46] Erol MK, Karakelleoglu S. Assessment of right heart function in the athlete's heart. Heart Vessels 2002;16(5):175–80.

[47] Pelliccia A, Maron BJ, Culasso F, et al. Athlete's heart in women: echocardiographic characterization of highly trained elite female athletes. JAMA 1996; 276:211–5.

[48] Montgomery HE, Clarkson P, Dollery CM, et al. Association of angiotensin-converting enzyme gene I/D polymorphism with change in left ventricular mass in response to physical training. Circulation 1997;96:741–7.

[49] Karjalainen J, Kujala UM, Stolt A, et al. Angiotensinogen gene M235T polymorphism predicts left ventricular hypertrophy in endurance athletes. J Am Coll Cardiol 1999;34(2):494–9.

[50] Pelliccia A, Thompson PD. The genetics of left ventricular remodeling in competitive athletes. J Cardiovasc Med 2006;7:267–70.

[51] Thomas LR, Douglas PS. Echocardiographic findings in athletes. In: Thompson PD, editor. Exercise and sports cardiology. New York: McGraw-Hill Companies; 2001. p. 43–70.

[52] Pelliccia A, Maron BJ, de Luca R, et al. Remodeling of left ventricular hypertrophy in elite athletes after long-term deconditioning. Circulation 2002;105: 944–9.

[53] Coyle EF, Martin WH 3rd, Sinacore DR, et al. Time course of loss of adaptations after stopping prolonged intense endurance training. J Appl Physiol 1984;57:1857–64.

[54] Maron BJ, Pelliccia A, Spataro A, et al. Reduction in left ventricular wall thickness after deconditioning in highly trained Olympic athletes. Br Heart J 1993; 69:125–8.

[55] Petersen SE, Selvanayagam JB, et al. Differentiation of athlete's heart from pathological forms of cardiac

hypertrophy by means of geometric indices derived from cardiovascular magnetic resonance. J Cardiovasc Magn Reson 2005;7(3):551–8.

[56] Scharhag J, Urhausan A, et al. No difference in N-terminal pro-brain natriuretic peptide (NT-proBNP) concentrations between endurance athletes with athlete's heart and healthy untrained controls. Heart 2004;90(9):1055–6.

[57] Maron BJ. Sudden death in young athletes. N Engl J Med 2003;349(11):1064–75.

[58] Thompson PD. The cardiovascular complications of vigorous physical activity. Arch Intern Med 1996; 156(20):2297–302.

[59] Maron BJ, Zipes DP. 36th Bethesda Conference: eligibility recommendations for competitive athletes with cardiovascular abnormalities. J Am Coll Cardiol 2005;45:1312–75.

[60] Mohlenkamp S, Lehmann N, Kiefer D, et al. Advanced-age marathon runners have a reduced Framingham risk score but their extent of coronary atherosclerosis is underestimated. Circulation 2006; 114(18, Suppl 2):II852.

[61] Lee IM, Skerett PJ. Physical activity and all-cause mortality: what is the dose-response relation? Med Sci Sports Exerc 2001;33(Suppl 6):S459–71.

[62] Maron BJ, Araujo CG, Thompson PD, et al. World Heart Federation; International Federation of Sports Medicine; American Heart Association Committee on Exercise, Cardiac Rehabilitation, and Prevention. Recommendations for preparticipation screening and the assessment of cardiovascular disease in master athletes: an advisory for healthcare professionals from the working groups of the World Heart Federation, the International Federation of Sports Medicine, and the American Heart Association Committee on Exercise, Cardiac Rehabilitation, and Prevention. Circulation 2001; 103(2):327–34.

ELSEVIER
SAUNDERS

Cardiol Clin 25 (2007) 383–389

CARDIOLOGY
CLINICS

The "Athlete's Heart": Relation to Gender and Race

F.M. Di Paolo, MD, Antonio Pelliccia, MD*

*Institute of Sport Medicine and Science, Italian National Olympic Committee,
Largo P. Gabrielli 1, Rome 00197, Italy*

Long-term athletic training is associated with changes in cardiac morphology, commonly described as "athlete's heart." Although numerous studies have investigated the effects of training on cardiac dimensions, most are limited to male Caucasian athletes, and few data are available regarding the effect of long-term exercise training on the woman's heart. One extensive study evaluated cardiac dimensions in 600 highly trained and elite female athletes compared with those of male teammates. In female athletes, left ventricular (LV) end-diastolic cavity dimension ranged from 40 to 66 mm (mean, 49 ± 4). The vast majority of female athletes showed absolute values within the normal limits (ie, end-diastolic diameter ≤ 54 mm), but a substantial minority (approximately 8%) had LV cavity size enlarged (diastolic dimension > 55 mm) and occasionally (1%) markedly dilated (ie, ≥ 60 mm). Maximal LV thickness ranged from 6 to 12 mm (mean, 8.2 ± 0.9) and was greater than 11 mm in a minority of female athletes (only 1.5%) but did not exceed the upper normal limits (ie, 12 mm), overlapping into an abnormal range (ie, ≥ 13 mm) compatible with hypertrophic cardiomyopathy in any female athlete. LV mass (normalized to body surface area) was 80 ± 16 g/m^2 and was greater than the accepted normal limits (ie, 110 g/m^2) in 6%. Few data have been published regarding the cardiac dimensions in athletes in relation to ethnic and race differences. It seems that a larger proportion of African American athletes compared with Caucasian athletes have an LV wall thickness exceeding upper

normal limits; finally, Asian athletes engaged in an extreme sport activity (such as ultra-marathon race) showed distinctly enlarged LV cardiac chambers.

Athlete's heart and gender

In the last two decades several studies have extensively described the cardiac dimensional changes associated with long-term athletic conditioning, ie, the "athlete's heart." Morphologic cardiac alterations in trained athletes include increased LV diastolic cavity dimension, wall thickness, and mass, which are considered physiologic adaptations to the hemodynamic load associated with chronic exercise training. Most studies investigating the "athlete's heart" have been limited to males athletes, however, and few data are available regarding the effect of long-term exercise training on the woman's heart. In recent years the increasing participation of women in a broader spectrum of athletic activities and their high level of achievement in competitions have raised attention to this issue and have prompted several studies investigating the woman's "athlete's heart" [1–5].

One of the most extensive studies published in this field evaluated 600 highly trained and elite female athletes [6]. This study took advantage of the database of the Institute of Sport Medicine and Science in Rome (Italy), where a large population of competitive athletes of both genders are serially examined with echocardiography as a part of the medical program implemented there [7]. The study included a cohort of 600 women who were free from structural cardiovascular disease and who were engaged in a wide range of 27 different sports with long-term participation in competitions, including approximately one third of

* Corresponding author.
E-mail address: antonio.pelliccia@coni.it
(A. Pelliccia).

whom were elite athletes who had recognition in World Championship and Olympic events.

Cardiac dimensions in female athletes

In the overall group of female athletes, LV end-diastolic cavity dimension ranged from 40 to 66 mm (mean, 49 ± 4 mm) (Fig. 1A). Although the vast majority of female athletes showed absolute values within the normal limits (ie, end-diastolic diameter ≤54 mm) [8], a substantial minority (approximately 8%) had LV cavity size enlarged (≥55 mm), and occasionally (1%) markedly dilated (ie, ≥60 mm). Maximal LV thickness (usually corresponding to the anterior ventricular septum) ranged from 6 to 12 mm (mean, 8.2 ± 0.9 mm). Maximum LV wall thickness was greater than 11 mm in a minority of female athletes (1.5%) and did not exceed the upper normal limits (ie, 12 mm) [8] in any of the 600 athletes. Finally, LV mass (normalized to body surface area) was 80±16 g/m^2 and was greater than the accepted normal limits (ie, 110 g/m^2) [9] in 6%.

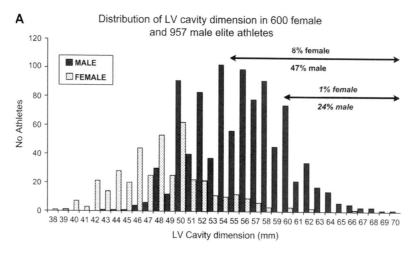

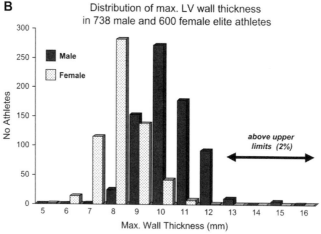

Fig. 1. (*A*) Distribution of maximum left ventricular cavity dimensions (end-diastolic diameter) in the 600 female athletes (*white bars with dots*). For comparison, distribution in a group of 957 male athletes of the same ethnic origin, age range, and spectrum of sport disciplines is shown (*gray bars*). Eight percent of female athletes exceed upper normal limits (ie, 54 mm) versus 47% of male athletes. Only four female athletes (1%) showed a particularly large chamber (≥60 mm) versus 179 male athletes (24%). (*B*) Distribution of maximum left ventricular wall thickness in 600 female athletes (*white bars with dots*). For comparison, distribution of maximum wall thickness in a group of 738 male athletes of the same ethnic origin, age range, and spectrum of sport disciplines is shown (*gray bars*). Although 2% of these athletes exceed upper normal limits (ie, 12 mm), women rarely have wall thickness greater than 11 mm and none exceed the normal limit.

Comparison of female athletes versus sedentary control subjects

When female athletes and sedentary female control subjects (of comparable age, body size, and racial composition) were compared, athletes showed enlarged LV cavity dimension (average, +6%), increased wall thickness (average, +14%), relative wall thickness (average, +9%), and mass normalized to body size (average, +25%). Compared with sedentary control subjects, athletes also showed mildly enlarged left atrial dimension (average, +4%) [6].

Despite morphologic differences, athletes did not show alterations of the indices of LV systolic function (ejection fraction was >50% in each); also, diastolic filling pattern as assessed by Doppler echocardiography was normal, including early diastolic peak flow velocity (73 ± 13 versus 72 ± 11 cm/sec in control subjects; p = not statistically significant) and deceleration of early peak flow velocity (521 ± 133 versus 515 ± 120 cm/sec^2 in control subjects; ns); however, late (atrial) peak flow velocity was lower in athletes than in control subjects (30 ± 8 versus 35 ± 8; $P<.001$) as a consequence of the lower heart rate typical of trained subjects. Consequently, athletes also showed increased ratio of the early to late peak flow velocities (2.6 ± 0.9 versus 2.2 ± 0.6 of control subjects; $P<.001$) [6].

More recently a study using cardiac magnetic resonance has included young adult elite female athletes, compared with age- and sex-matched sedentary control subjects [10]. This study confirms that female athletes showed increased left and right ventricular volumes and mass when compared with control subjects (ranging from +15% to +50%). In particular athletes showed LV end-diastolic volume index 94 ± 9 versus 80 ± 10 mL/m^2 in sedentary control subjects and LV mass index 70 ± 9 versus 52 ± 9 g/m^2 in control subjects [10].

Comparison of female versus male elite athletes

In a previous analysis the authors used a group of 738 male athletes [11] of similar age, ethnic origin, sporting disciplines, and intensity of training, for comparison with the group of 600 female athletes [6]. Elite female athletes when compared with elite male athletes showed smaller absolute LV cavity dimension (−11%), maximum wall thickness (−23%), relative wall thickness (−9%), and mass normalized to body size (−31%). Also, dimensions of aortic root (−9%) and left atrial chamber (−14%) were smaller in female athletes (Table 1).

Table 1
Cardiac dimensions in athletes in relation to gender

	Female athletes (mean±SD)	Male athletes (mean±SD)	$P<$	Reference
LVDD (mm)	48.9 ± 4.0	54.2 ± 4.0	.001	[6]
	8% ≥55	47% ≥55		
	49.6 ± 3.1	54.1 ± 4.1	.001	[24]
	None >60	5.8% >60		
	47.7 ± 3.3	51.6 ± 3.3	.001	[25]
	47.7 ± 3.3	54.1 ± 4.1	.001	[27]
	None ≥55	11% ≥55		
WT (mm)	8.2 ± 0.9	10.1 ± 1.2	.001	[6]
	0% >12	2% >12		
	8.7 ± 1.2	10.4 ± 1.5	.001	[24]
	0% >12	2.5% >12		
	8.4 ± 1.1	9.8 ± 1.2	.001	[25]
	None >12	0.4% >12		
LV mass (g)	133 ± 32	206 ± 46	.001	[6]
	190 ± 41	269 ± 63	.001	[24]
	160 ± 50	211 ± 65	.001	[25]

Abbreviations: LV, left ventricular; LVDD, left ventricular diastolic dimensions; WT, wall thickness.

LV cavity size in female athletes showed a wide range of values, from 40 to 66 mm, which was similar to that observed in male athletes (ie, from 44 to 66 mm). In contrast, LV wall thickness showed a broader range of values in male (7 to 16 mm) than in female (6 to 12 mm) athletes [12]. Indeed, LV wall thickness exceeded the upper limits of normal in a small subset of elite male athletes (2%), whereas it remained within the accepted normal limits in all female athletes (Fig. 1).

The gender-related differences in LV wall thickness were not completely explained by the different body size (or composition) of the female athletes, because normalization of LV wall thickness for body surface area (or height) did not abolish differences among sexes, and men continued to significantly exceed women [6]. Other studies [10,11] evaluating selected groups of male and female athletes, however, have not been able to confirm gender-related differences in left and right ventricular volumes.

Determinants of left ventricular remodeling in female athletes

The authors assessed the impact of potential determinants on LV dimensions by stepwise regression analysis in the group of 600 athletes previously described [6]. The authors found that approximately 50% of the variability in LV cavity dimension was associated with body size, increasing age, and lower resting heart rate (which in this population also reflects the duration and intensity of athletic conditioning). Analysis of covariance confirmed the independent impact of type of sport and showed that endurance disciplines, such as cycling, cross country skiing, and rowing/canoeing had the greatest effect (ie, enlargement) on LV cavity dimensions. Other disciplines, such as soccer, basketball, handball, and other team ball sports (which include aerobic and anaerobic exercise training) showed a moderate impact on LV cavity dimension; finally, technical disciplines such as equestrian or yachting had only a minimal effect on cardiac dimensions (Fig. 2).

These findings are consistent with similar analysis previously performed in male athletes, in which different training profiles have been shown to alter cardiac dimensions in a different fashion, with endurance disciplines demonstrating the greatest impact on LV cavity dimension and wall thickness as it occurs in female athletes [11].

It is also possible that other factors may explain part of the gender-related cardiac dimensional differences. Although a large proportion of the differences between males and females seems to be related to different body size, other mechanisms implicated are the lower increase in absolute blood pressure during peak exercise in women [13] and their lower level of natural androgenic hormones, which stimulates cardiac protein synthesis [14]. Finally, genetic factors have recently achieved greater recognition as independent determinants in the cardiac remodeling of trained athletes [15–17].

Outer limits of left ventricular remodeling in female athletes and implications for cardiovascular screening

The upper limits to which absolute LV dimensions are increased as a consequence of athletic conditioning in women have particular relevance to the differential diagnosis between "athlete's heart" and structural cardiovascular

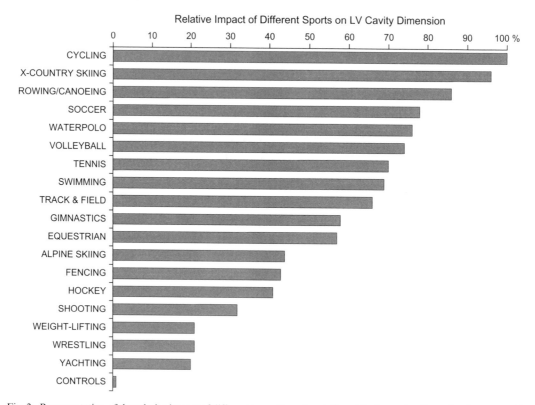

Fig. 2. Representation of the relative impact of different type of sport on left ventricular cavity dimension (as assessed by stepwise and covariance analysis) in a population of 600 competitive female athletes [6]. The impact of each type of sport is shown in comparison with others, given that the impact of sedentary matched control subjects is equal to zero. Hockey, field hockey.

disease. In fact, female athletes not uncommonly show enlarged LV cavity dimension (ie, end-diastolic dimension ≥ 54 mm) and occasionally markedly dilated dimension (≥ 60 mm) that overlaps into a distinctively pathologic range observed in patients who have dilated cardiomyopathy (DCM) [18,19]. This morphologic finding raises a differential diagnosis between an extreme physiologic adaptation to intensive exercise training and a pathologic cardiac condition such as DCM, with the potential for adverse clinical consequences. Resolution of this dilemma has relevant clinical and legal consequences, because the correct identification of the physiologic nature of LV dilatation may avoid an unnecessary withdrawal of the athlete from competitions and the unjustified loss of the varied benefits (including economic) derived from the sport [20].

Certain criteria have been suggested to help in this differential diagnosis: in patients who have DCM, the LV cavity is disproportionately enlarged and modifies to a more spherical shape [19]; in trained athletes, LV cavity enlargement is associated with consistent enlargement of the right ventricle; indeed, the physiologically dilated LV cavity maintains the ellipsoid shape, with the mitral valve normally positioned and without mitral regurgitation [21,22]. The most definitive evidence for DCM is, however, the presence of global systolic dysfunction (ie, ejection fraction $<50\%$) or evidence of segmental wall motion abnormalities. Instead, athletes with physiologic LV cavity enlargement do not show global or segmental systolic dysfunction or abnormal diastolic filling or relaxation [21]. Finally, LV cavity enlargement is a common finding in athletes engaged in largely aerobic disciplines, such as cycling, cross-country skiing, rowing, and long-distance running, and is usually associated with a superior physical performance [21].

The upper limits of absolute LV wall thickness in female athletes rarely exceeds 11 mm and unlikely overlaps into the abnormal range (ie, ≥ 13 mm) compatible with hypertrophic cardiomyopathy (HCM) [23]. This observation seems to differ significantly from that found in male athletes, in whom LV wall thicknesses may exceed upper normal limits (ie, 12 mm) in a significant minority [11,24,25]. Intense athletic conditioning therefore apparently does not represent a sufficient stimulus to increase LV wall thicknesses in women up to the gray zone of borderline LV hypertrophy, and such athletes do not show morphologic changes that resemble HCM [6]. Considering that male and female patients who have HCM show a similar magnitude of LV wall thickening [26], the presence of LV wall thickness of greater than or equal to 13 mm in a female athlete is unlikely to represent a physiologic consequence of athletic conditioning and more likely is an expression of a primary pathologic hypertrophy, such as HCM.

A more recent study performed in elite male and female British athletes also supports these results [24]: 442 adult elite athletes engaged in 13 different sports were profiled with echocardiography; of these 136 were female. None of the female athletes showed maximum LV wall thickness greater than 11 mm; LV diameter was less than or equal to 60 mm in all athletes. Systolic and diastolic function were within normal limits for all athletes and similar to those observed in control subjects.

Finally, in a population of highly trained adolescent athletes examined by Makan and colleagues [27] the upper limits of LV cavity were found to be smaller than in adults; the LV cavity size exceeded normal limits (ie, >54 mm) in 18% of 900 athletes, and most of them (77%) were males.

Athlete's heart and race

Cardiac dimensions in relation to race

Clinical evidence suggests that racial differences may exist in the response to certain cardiovascular pathologic conditions, such as systemic hypertension. For example, it is recognized that Afro-Caribbean hypertensive patients show a more substantial increase in LV mass than do Caucasian individuals [28]. It is, therefore, possible that the increased preload or afterload and mean systolic blood pressure associated with prolonged exercise training may give rise to more marked morphologic cardiac changes in Afro-Caribbean compared with Caucasian athletes. Few data are available, however, describing the physiologic cardiac adaptation to athletic conditioning in African, Afro-Caribbean, and African American populations.

In a study of African American athletes, Lewis and colleagues [29] evaluated 265 (99% black) collegiate athletes as part of a screening program to identify occult cardiac disease. In this study, 13% of African American athletes had an left ventricular wall thickness (LVWT) of greater than 12 mm and 1.1% had an LVWT of 16 to 18 mm. All these individuals were normotensive and denied

Table 2
Cardiac dimensions in athletes in relation to race

	African American athletes [29] n=265	West African athletes [31] n=21	Asian athletes [34] n=291	Caucasian athletes [21] n=1309
LVDD (mm)	52±4 (11% >55)	54.1±4.2	61.8±6.9	55.5±4.3 (45% >55)
WT (mm)	11±2 (11% >12)	10.6±1.2 None >12	10.2±1.9	9.3±1.4 (1.1% >12)
Ao (mm)	31±3	29.6±3.6	38.5±4.0	33.3±2.6
LA (mm)	36±4	38.2±4.6	40.2±4.8	35±4
LV mass (g)	202±56	261±28	nd	181±62

Abbreviations: Ao, aortic root; LA, left atrium; LV, left ventricular; LVDD, left ventricular diastolic dimensions; WT, wall thickness; nd, no data.

drug abuse (but formal drug testing was not performed). In this study, therefore, 13% of athletes had an LVWT exceeding the upper normal limits, a finding that is different from the authors' experience with Caucasian athletes, in whom only 2% showed LVWT greater than 12 mm [11]. Although it is unlikely that 13% of African American athletes represent true HCM (the prevalence of the disease in the general population, including African Americans, is 0.2%) [30], it is possible that LV hypertrophy in these athletes represents a marked cardiac response to physical training.

Data on African athletes are lacking: only one recent investigation has assessed the cardiac dimensional changes in a group of highly trained Cameroonian handball players; it showed an increase of LV cavity size, mass, wall thickness, and left atrial diameter in athletes in comparison with sedentary control subjects (age-, sex-, height-, and weight-matched) [31].

Finally, in a population of 140 elite African/Afro-Caribbean athletes recently examined by Sharma, the average LV wall thickness was reported to be 9.6% higher in African and Afro-Caribbean athletes compared with 170 matched Caucasian athletes (11.1 versus 10.0 mm; $P < .001$), and 20% of the African athletes showed wall thickness exceeding upper normal limits (ie, ≥ 12 mm) (Table 2) [32].

The exact stimulus to the disproportionate LV wall thickening in response to exercise training observed in African American athletes remains unknown; however, an increased blood pressure response to exercise has been demonstrated in African American athletes [33], which provides one possible mechanism for the differences between black and white athletes. More systematic studies are, however, required to define the presence of a marked LV response to exercise training and the upper physiologic limits of cardiac dimensions in African, African American, and Afro-Caribbean athletes.

Only few data have been published regarding the cardiac dimensions in Asian athletes [34]. In a group of 291 Japanese participants in an extreme sport activity, such as the 100-km ultra-marathon, LV end-diastolic diameter was reported to be markedly enlarged (61.8 ± 6.9 mm; range, 42–75 mm), the average septal thickness was within normal limits (10.2 ± 1.4 mm; range, 5–19 mm) and so was the posterior wall thickness (10.0 ± 1.4 mm; range, 5–15 mm), but the left atrial diameter was mildly enlarged (40.2 ± 4.8 mm; range, 26–49 mm). In this special subset of athletes, 33 (11%) had LV diastolic diameter greater than or equal to 70 mm, and the investigators reported that some athletes also had markedly enlarged aortic root and left atrium more than had ever been previously reported [35]. Although the influence of genetic and racial determinants cannot be excluded, the extreme hemodynamic demand of the ultra-marathon makes this special subset of Japanese population unsuitable for race-related comparison.

References

[1] Pluim BM, Zwinderman AH, van der Laarse A, et al. A meta-analysis of cardiac structure and function. Circulation 1999;100:336–44.
[2] Huston TP, Puffer JC, Rodney WM. The athletic heart syndrome. N Engl J Med 1985;4:24–32.
[3] Maron BJ. Structural features of the athlete heart as defined by echocardiography. J Am Coll Cardiol 1986;7:190–203.
[4] Spirito P, Pelliccia A, Proschan M, et al. Morphology of the "athlete's heart" assessed by echocardiography in 947 elite athletes representing 27 sports. Am J Cardiol 1994;74:802–6.
[5] Fagard R. Athlete's heart. Heart 2003;89:1455–61.

[6] Pelliccia A, Maron BJ, Culasso F, et al. The athlete's heart in women: echocardiographic characterization of 600 highly trained and elite female athletes. JAMA 1996;276:211–5.

[7] Pelliccia A, Maron BJ. Preparticipation cardiovascular evaluation of the competitive athlete: perspectives from the 30-year Italian experience. Am J Cardiol 1995;75:827–9.

[8] Henry WL, Gardin JM, Ware JH. Echocardiographic measurements in normal subjects from infancy to old age. Circulation 1980;62:1054–61.

[9] Gardin JM, Savage DD, Ware JH, et al. Effect of age, sex, body surface area on echocardiographic left ventricular wall mass in normal subjects. Hypertension 1987;9(Suppl II):II36–9.

[10] Petersen SE, Hudsmith LE, Robson MD, et al. Sex-specific characteristics of cardiac function, geometry, and mass in young adult elite athletes. J Magn Reson Imaging 2006;24(2):297–303.

[11] Pelliccia A, Maron BJ, Spataro A, et al. The upper limit of physiologic cardiac hypertrophy in highly trained elite athletes. N Engl J Med 1991;324:295–301.

[12] Legaz-Arrese A, Gonzalez-Cerretero M, Lacambra-Blasco I. Adaptation of left ventricular morphology to long-term training in sprint- and endurance-trained elite runners. Eur J Appl Physiol 2006; 96(6):740–6.

[13] Gleim GW, Stachenfeld NS, Coplan NL, et al. Gender differences in the systolic blood pressure response to exercise. Am Heart J 1991;121:524–30.

[14] McGill HC, Anselmo VC, Buchanan JM, et al. The heart is a target for androgen. Science 1980;207: 775–7.

[15] Montgomery HE, Clarkson P, Dollery CM, et al. Association of angiotensin-converting enzyme gene I/D polymorphism with change in left ventricular mass in response to physical training. Circulation 1997;96:741–7.

[16] Karjalainen J, Kujala HM, Stolt A, et al. Angiotensinogen gene M235T polymorphism predicts left ventricular hypertrophy in endurance athletes. J Am Coll Cardiol 1999;34:494–9.

[17] Pelliccia A, Thompson PD. The genetics of left ventricular remodeling in competitive athletes. J Cardiovasc Med 2006;7(4):267–70.

[18] Manolio TA, Baughman KL, Rodeheffer R, et al. Prevalence and etiology of idiopathic dilated cardiomyopathy. Am J Cardiol 1992;69:1458–66.

[19] Gavazzi A, De Maria R, Renosto G, et al. The spectrum of left ventricular size in dilated cardiomyopathy: clinical correlates and prognostic implications. Am Heart J 1993;125:410–42.

[20] Maron BJ, Zipes DP. 36th Bethesda Conference: eligibility recommendations for competitive athletes with cardiovascular abnormalities. J Am Coll Cardiol 2005;45:2–64.

[21] Pelliccia A, Culasso F, Di Paolo FM, et al. Physiologic left ventricular cavity dilatation in elite athletes. Ann Intern Med 1999;130:23–31.

[22] Pelliccia A, Avelar E, De Castro S, et al. Global left ventricular shape is not altered as a consequence of physiologic remodeling in highly trained athletes. Am J Cardiol 2000;86:700–2.

[23] Maron BJ. Hypertrophic cardiomyopathy: a systematic review. JAMA 2002;287:1308–20.

[24] Whyte GP, George K, Sharma S, et al. The upper limit of physiological cardiac hypertrophy in elite male and female athletes: the British experience. Eur J Appl Physiol 2004;92:592–7.

[25] Sharma S, Maron BJ, Whyte G, et al. Physiologic limits of left ventricular hypertrophy in elite junior athletes: relevance to differential diagnosis of athlete's heart and hypertrophic cardiomyopathy. J Am Coll Cardiol 2002;1431–6.

[26] Klues HG, Schiffers A, Maron BJ. Phenotypic spectrum and patterns of left ventricular hypertrophy in hypertrophic cardiomyopathy: morphologic observations and significance as assessed by two-dimensional echocardiography in 600 patients. J Am Coll Cardiol 1995;26:1699–708.

[27] Makan J, Sharma S, Firooz S, et al. Physiological upper limits of ventricular cavity size in highly trained adolescent athletes. Heart 2005;91:495–9.

[28] Dunn FG, Oigman W, Sungaard-Riise K, et al. Racial differences in cardiac adaptation to essential hypertension determined by echocardiographic indexes. J Am Coll Cardiol 1983;1:1348–51.

[29] Lewis J, Maron B, Diggs J, et al. Pre participation echocardiographic screening for cardiovascular disease in a large, predominantly black population of college athletes. Am J Cardiol 1989;64:1029–33.

[30] Maron BJ, Gardin JM, Flack JM, et al. Prevalence of hypertrophic cardiomyopathy in a general population of young adults: echocardiographic analysis of 4111 subjects in the CARDIA study. Coronary artery risk development in (young) adults. Circulation 1995;785–9.

[31] Dzudie A, Menanga A, Hamadou B, et al. Ultrasonographic study of left ventricular function at rest in a group of highly trained black African handball players. Eur J Echocardiogr 2006;8(2):122–7.

[32] Basavarajaiah S, Carby L, Wilson M, et al. Left ventricular remodeling in highly trained black athletes of African/Afro-Caribbean origin. Eur J Cardiovasc Prev Rehab 2007;14(1):S108.

[33] Ekelund LG, Suchindran CM, Karon JM, et al. Black–white differences in exercise blood pressure. The Lipid Research Clinics Program Prevalence Study. Circulation 1990;81:1568–74.

[34] Nagashima J, Musha H, Takada H, et al. New upper limit of physiologic cardiac hypertrophy in Japanese participants in the 100-km ultramarathon. J Am Coll Cardiol 2003;42:1617–23.

[35] Pelliccia BJ, Maron FM, Di Paolo A, et al. Prevalence and clinical significance of left atrial remodeling in competitive athletes. J Am Coll Cardiol 2005;46(4):690–6.

ELSEVIER
SAUNDERS

CARDIOLOGY
CLINICS

Cardiol Clin 25 (2007) 391–397

How to Screen Athletes for Cardiovascular Diseases

Domenico Corrado, MD, PhD[a,*], Pierantonio Michieli, MD, PhD[b],
Cristina Basso, MD, PhD[c], Maurizio Schiavon, MD[b],
Gaetano Thiene, MD, FRCP Hon[c]

[a]Division of Cardiology, Department of Cardiac, Thoracic and Vascular Sciences,
University of Padova Medical School, Via Giustiniani 2, 35121 Padova, Italy
[b]Center for Sports Medicine and Physical Activity Unit, Social Health Department,
ULSS 16, via dei Colli 4, 35143 Padova, Italy
[c]Cardiovascolar Pathology, Department of Medical-Diagnostic Sciences,
University of Padova Medical School, via Gabelli 61, 35121 Padova, Italy

The majority of athletes who die suddenly have previously unsuspected structural heart diseases [1–10]. The causes of sudden cardiac death (SCD) reflect the age of participants. In older athletes (adults over 35 years), atherosclerotic coronary artery disease is the most common cause of fatalities. In young athletes, there is a broad spectrum of cardiovascular substrates, including congenital and inherited heart disorders (Box 1). Cardiomyopathies have been consistently implicated as the leading cause of sports-related cardiac arrest in the young, with hypertrophic cardiomyopathy (HCM) accounting for more than one third of fatal cases in the United States [1,3,7,9] and arrhythmogenic right ventricular cardiomyopathy (ARVC) for approximately one fourth in Italy [2,4–6,10].

The most common mechanism of SCD in young competitive athletes is abrupt ventricular fibrillation as a consequence of these underlying cardiovascular diseases. The culprit diseases are often clinically silent and unlikely to be suspected or diagnosed on the basis of spontaneous symptoms [1–5]. Preparticipation medical evaluation of athletic populations offers the ability to identify asymptomatic athletes who have potentially lethal cardiovascular abnormalities, and to protect them from the risk of SCD through disqualification from competitive sports [5,8]. This article addresses the efficacy and feasibility of preparticipation screening, essentially based on 12-lead ECG, as has been in practice in Italy for 25 years.

Italian screening protocol

Italy is the only country in the world where preparticipation evaluation is required by law. A mass screening program, essentially based on 12-lead ECG, has been the practice for 25 years. Fig. 1 [5,6] reports the flow chart of the Italian protocol for cardiovascular screening of young competitive athletes. First-line examination includes family history, physical examination, and 12-lead ECG. Additional tests are requested only for subjects who have positive findings at initial evaluation. Athletes diagnosed with cardiovascular diseases are managed according to available guidelines. Screening usually starts at the beginning of competitive athletic activity (age 12–14 years) and is repeated on a regular basis. Screening in children is not justified because the phenotypic manifestations—both ECG abnormalities and arrhythmic substrates—of most inherited heart diseases associated with risk for SCD are age-dependent and occur during adolescence and young adulthood [10].

12-lead ECG makes the difference

SCD during sports is most often the first clinical manifestation of an underlying

---

* Corresponding author.
  E-mail address: domenico.corrado@unipd.it
(D. Corrado).

Box 1. Cardiovascular causes of sudden death associated with sports

Age greater than or equal to 35 years
  Atherosclerotic coronary artery disease
Age less than 35 years
  Hypertrophic cardiomyopathy
  Arrhythmogenic right ventricular cardiomyopathy or dysplasia
  Premature coronary atherosclerosis
  Congenital anomalies of coronary arteries
  Myocarditis
  Aortic rupture
  Valvular disease
  Pre-excitation syndromes and conduction diseases
  Ion channel diseases
  Congenital heart disease, operated or unoperated

cardiovascular disease, which is usually clinically silent. This explains why a screening protocol based solely on the athlete's history and physical examination is of limited value for identification of athletes at risk for SCD. Preparticipation cardiovascular screening has traditionally been performed in the United States by means of history (personal and family) and physical examination, without 12-lead ECG or other testing, which are requested largely at the discretion of the examining physician [1,7]. This screening method has been recommended by the American Heart Association Council on Nutrition, Physical Activity, and Metabolism on the assumption that 12-lead ECG is not cost-effective for screening large populations of young athletes because of its low specificity [7]. The United States screening strategy, however, has a limited power to detect potentially lethal cardiovascular abnormalities in young athletes. One retrospective analysis in the United States, on 134 high school and collegiate athletes who died suddenly, showed that cardiovascular

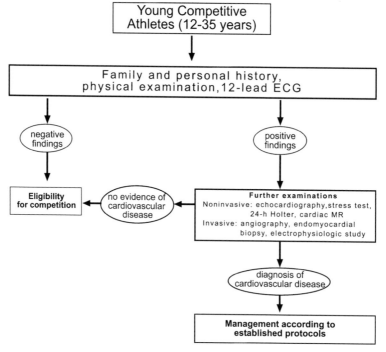

Fig. 1. Flow chart showing the protocol for cardiovascular screening of young competitive athletes that has been in practice in Italy for 25 years. MR, magnetic resonance. (*Modified from* Corrado D, Pelliccia A, Bjørnstad HH, et al. Cardiovascular preparticipation screening of young competitive athletes for prevention of sudden death: proposal for a common european protocol. Consensus statement of the Study Group of Sport Cardiology of the Working Group of Cardiac Rehabilitation and Exercise Physiology and the Working Group of Myocardial and Pericardial Diseases of the European Society of Cardiology. Eur Heart J 2005;26:516–24; with permission.)

abnormalities were suspected by standard history and physical examination screening only in 3% of the examined athletes and, eventually, less than 1% received an accurate diagnosis [11].

The addition of 12-lead ECG has the potential to enhance the sensitivity of the screening process for detection of cardiovascular diseases at risk for sudden death. In fact, ECG is abnormal in up to 95% of patients with HCM [1,6], which is the leading cause of sudden death athletes. Likewise, ECG abnormalities have also been documented in the majority of athletes who died from ARVC, proven at autopsy [4–6,12]. Moreover, 12-lead ECG offers the potential to detect (or to raise clinical suspicion) other potentially lethal conditions manifesting with ECG abnormalities, such as dilated cardiomyopathy, Wolff-Parkinson-White syndrome, Lènegre conduction disease, long and short QT syndromes, and Brugada syndrome. Based on published series either from the United States or Italy, these cardiomyopathies, cardiac conduction diseases, and channelopathies account for up to 60% of sudden deaths in young competitive athletes [1,5,13]. The possibility of detecting either premature coronary atherosclerosis or anomalous coronary artery in young competitive athletes is limited by the scarcity of baseline ECG signs of myocardial ischemia. However, the authors reported that approximately one fourth of young athletes who died of coronary artery diseases had warning symptoms or ECG abnormalities at preparticipation screening that could have raised suspicion of cardiac disease [5].

Comparison between the Italian screening protocol and that recommended by the American Heart Association demonstrates that 12-lead ECG makes the difference [14]. Among the 33,735 young competitive athletes screened in the Padua country area, a potentially lethal cardiovascular disease was actually detected in 43 athletes (0.13%) and consisted of HCM in 22, ARVC in 8, dilated cardiomyopathy in 4, Marfan syndrome in 3, long QT syndrome in 2, premature coronary artery disease in 2, myocarditis in 1, and subvalvular aortic stenosis in 1. Only 10 (23%) of these 43 athletes had a positive family history, an abnormal physical examination, or both at preparticipation evaluation that would have allowed their detection according to the American Heart Association protocol. Accordingly, the estimated sensitivity of screening modality based on 12-lead ECG for identification of athletes at risk for SCD is 77% greater than that of the screening protocol recommended by the American Heart Association.

Appropriate interpretation of an athlete's ECG saves lives as well as money

The 25-year Italian experience has demonstrated the crucial importance of appropriate interpretation of ECG abnormalities for proper cardiovascular evaluation and management of young competitive athletes [6,15]. Preparticipation evaluation of Italian athletes is performed by physicians who have specific training, medical skill, and scientific background to reliably identify relevant familial history, clinical symptoms, and ECG abnormalities. Physicians primarily responsible for screening and determination of eligibility for competitive sports attend postgraduate residency training programs in sports medicine (and sports cardiology) on a full-time basis for 4 years. These specialists work in sports medical centers specifically devoted to periodic evaluation of athletes.

Misinterpretation of ECG by nonexperienced physicians may lead to serious consequences [15]. Athletes may undergo an expensive diagnostic work-up or may be unnecessarily disqualified from competition for abnormalities, such as isolated voltage criteria for left ventricular hypertrophy (LVH), that fall within the normal range for athletes. Conversely, signs of potentially lethal organic heart disease, such as T-wave inversion, may be misinterpreted as normal variants of an athlete's ECG. The experience of screening athletes for HCM and ARVC/D is noteworthy in this regard.

The majority of patients with HCM have an abnormal ECG, with repolarization changes, pathologic Q waves, and left axis deviation being the commonest findings [5,16,17]. Isolated QRS voltage criteria for left ventricular hypertrophy (Sokolow-Lyon or Cornell criteria) is an unusual pattern in patients with HCM, in whom pathologic hypertrophy is characteristically associated with additional ECG abnormalities, such as left atrial enlargement, left axis deviation, delayed intrinsicoid deflection, T-wave inversion in inferior, anterior, or lateral leads, and pathologic Q waves [5,16–18]. Such ECG abnormalities of HCM need to be clearly distinguished from the ECG patterns seen in trained athletes in whom physiologic hypertrophy manifests as an isolated increase of QRS amplitude, with right QRS axis deviation, normal atrial and ventricular activation patterns, and normal ST-T repolarization [18–22].

The authors recently examined and compared the ECG tracings of 260 consecutive patients with clinical and echocardiographic diagnosis of HCM, and those of 1,005 trained athletes undergoing preparticipation cardiovascular evaluation, including ECG and echocardiography [17,19,23]. An ECG abnormality was found in 246 out of 260 (94.6%) patients with HCM, and in 817 of 1,005 athletes (81.3%). The majority of patients with HCM had one or more of the following ECG changes: repolarization ST/T abnormalities in 209 (80%), pathologic Q waves in 103 (39.6%), left atrial enlargement in 75 (28.8%), intraventricular conduction abnormalities in 71 (27.3%), and left axis deviation in 9 (3.5%). ECG tracings showed isolated increase of QRS voltages in only 5 HCM patients (1.9%) and were completely normal in 14 (5.4%).

Compared with patients with HCM, trained athletes significantly more often had isolated voltage criteria for LVH (403, or 40%), but significantly less often negative T waves (27, or 2.7%), pathologic Q waves (17, or 1.7%), and nonvoltage criteria of LVH (13, or 1.3%). No athletes with isolated voltage criteria had echocardiographic evidence of HCM. This study shows that ECG of HCM overlaps marginally with ECG findings in trained athletes. An isolated increase of QRS voltage is an unusual pattern (1.9%) of LVH in patients with HCM, while it is frequently observed (40%) in trained athletes. Thus, systematic echocardiographic evaluation of athletes fulfilling isolated QRS voltage criteria at preparticipation screening is not justified, unless such subjects have other ECG changes suggesting pathologic LVH, relevant symptoms, abnormal physical examination, or a positive family history for cardiovascular diseases or premature SCD, therefore resulting in a considerable cost savings.

There is a general misconception that inverted T-waves in precordial leads are frequently encountered in trained athletes, being part of the spectrum of cardiovascular adaptive changes to physical exercise [18]. In particular, T-wave inversion in right precordial leads (beyond V1) is often dismissed in young competitive athletes as non-specific or as persistence of the juvenile T-wave pattern. Detailed analysis of available data shows that the prevalence of T-wave inversion in two or more precordial leads did not exceed 4% in large athletic populations (age equal to or more than 14 years), regardless of training intensity and duration; moreover, there does not seem to be a greater prevalence in trained athletes as compared with sedentary people [24,25]. On the other

hand, T-wave inversion is an important ECG marker of cardiomyopathies, cardiac ion channellopathies, ischemic heart disease, and aortic valve disease [6]. Of note, right precordial T-wave inversion is present in up to 87% of patients who have ARVC, a recognized leading cause of athletic field sudden death worldwide [5,6,12]. Recently, the authors assessed prospectively the prevalence and clinical significance of T-wave abnormality in right precordial leads on the basal 12-lead ECG of 3,086 consecutive young competitive athletes who underwent preparticipation screening at the Center for Sports Medicine in Padua [26]. One hundred-twenty seven athletes (4.1%) showed T-wave inversion beyond V1. The prevalence of right precordial T-wave inversion decreased significantly with increasing age (1.4% in athletes aged more than or equal to 14 years, versus 9.3% in those aged less than 14 years), body surface area, and body mass index; moreover, it was significantly lower in individuals with complete versus incomplete pubertal development (1.3% versus 10.5%). There was no statistically significant association between right precordial T-wave inversion and gender, type of sports, and level of athletic training. Among the 127 athletes who underwent ecocardiographic study because of right precordial T-wave inversion, three (2.3%) were diagnosed with ARVC/D and disqualified from competitive sports activity, accounting for an estimated disease prevalence of 0.1% in the general young athletic population.

Thus, T-wave inversion in right precordial leads is an uncommon ECG finding in postpubertal athletes and deserves accurate investigation because it may reflect an underlying ARVC/D. The athlete with right precordial T-wave inversion should be thoroughly investigated by imaging techniques, exercise test and 24-hour Holter monitoring and, when possible, by genetic testing to exclude a pathologic basis. Genotype-phenotype correlation studies in cardiomyopathy reveal that ECG abnormalities can represent the only sign of disease expression in mutation carriers, even in the absence of any other features, or before structural changes in the heart can be detected [27]. Accordingly, the perspective that T-wave inversion is caused by cardiovascular adaptation in an athlete should only be accepted once inherited forms of cardiovascular disease have been definitively excluded by a comprehensive clinical work-up, including investigation of family members.

Efficacy of preparticpation screening

The Italian long-term experience has provided compelling evidence of screening efficacy in identifying athletes at risk for SCD and in preventing SCD. Among 33,735 athletes undergoing preparticipation screening at the Center for Sport Medicine in Padua, 22 (0.07%) showed definitive evidence, both clinical and echocardiographic, of HCM. An absolute value of screening sensitivity for HCM cannot be derived from these data because systematic echocardiographic findings were not available. However, the 0.07% prevalence of HCM found in the white athletic population of the Veneto region of Italy, evaluated by history, physical examination, and ECG, is similar to the 0.10% prevalence reported for young white individuals in the United States, as assessed by echocardiography. This finding indicates that the Italian screening, which is essentially based on 12-lead ECG, may be as sensitive as echocardiographic screening in detecting HCM in the young athletic population.

These results were confirmed by Pelliccia and colleagues [28]. In their study, 4,450 members of Italian national teams, initially judged eligible for competition as a result of Italian baseline systematic preparticipation screening (ie, history, physical examination, and 12-lead ECG), subsequently underwent clinical and echocardiographic examination at the Institute of Sports Sciences in Rome to assess for the presence of undetected hypertrophic cardiomyopathy or other structural cardiac disease. None of the 4,450 athletes showed evidence of hypertrophic cardiomyopathy. This study further demonstrates that Italian national preparticipation screening programs, including 12-lead ECG, is efficient in identifying athletes with hypertrophic cardiomyopathy, and that echocardiography does not increase screening sensitivity.

The final objective of screening athletes for cardiovascular diseases is to prevent SCD during sports. There is growing evidence that that systematic preparticipation screening using ECG is a lifesaving strategy. None of the 22 young athletes with HCM who were identified by preparticipation athletic screening in the Padua country area, and were disqualified from training and competition, died during an average 8-year follow-up period [5]. This favorable long-term outcome of former athletes with HCM was the result not only of restriction from competitive sports activity, but also of the subsequent close

follow-up and clinical management aimed at preventing SCD. These findings indicate that preparticipation screening does not change merely the mode of death from exercise-related to exercise-unrelated, but actually reduces mortality from HCM.

A time-trend analysis of the incidence of SCD in young competitive athletes aged 12 to 35 years in the Veneto region of Italy, between 1979 and 2004, confirmed and extended the authors' previous observations in athletes with HCM [29]. The long-term impact of the screening program on prevention of SCD during sports was assessed by comparing temporal trends in sudden death among screened athletes and unscreened nonathletes. Assessed intervals were prescreening (1979–1981), early screening (1982–1992), and late screening (1993–2004). During the entire study period, in unscreened nonathletes, the incidence of SCD was steady at about 0.8 per 100,000 person-years; in contrast, the SCD rates in screened athletes declined from 4.2 per 100,000 person-years in the prescreening interval, to 2.4 in early-screening, and to 0.9 in late-screening (Fig. 2). Most of the reduction was attributable to fewer deaths from HCM and ARVC. A parallel study of disqualifications from competitive sports at the Center for Sports Medicine in the Padua country area showed that the proportion of athletes identified and disqualified for cardiomyopathies doubled from the early to the late screening period [29]. This indicates that mortality reduction was a reflection of a lower incidence of sudden death from cardiomyopathies, as a result of increasing identification over time of affected athletes at preparticipation screening.

Screening feasibility and cost-effectiveness

The long-term Italian experience shows that screening is made feasible because of its limited costs in the setting of a mass-program. The cost of performing a preparticipation cardiac history and physical examination by qualified physicians has been estimated to be 25 Euro per athlete, and rises to 40 Euro per athlete if a 12-lead ECG is added. The screening cost is covered by the athlete or by the athletic team, except for athletes younger than 18 years, for whom the expense is supported by the National Health System [6].

The cost of further evaluation of athletes with positive findings at first-line examination is smaller than expected on the basis of the

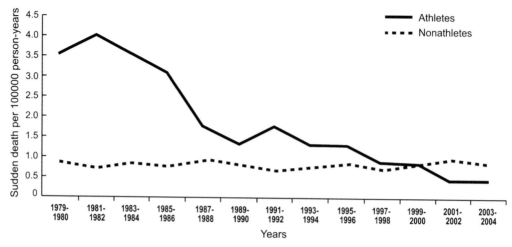

Fig. 2. Annual incidence rates of SCD per 100,000 persons, among screened competitive athletes and unscreened non-athletes 12 to 35 years of age in the Veneto Region of Italy, from 1979 to 2004. During the study period (the nationwide preparticipation screening program was launched in 1982), the annual incidence of SCD declined by 89% in screened athletes (P for trend <0.001). In contrast, the incidence rate of SCD did not demonstrate consistent changes over time in unscreened nonathletes. (*Modified from* Corrado D, Basso C, Pavei A, et al. Trends in sudden cardiovascular death in young competitive athletes after implementation of a preparticipation screening program. JAMA 2006;296:1593–601; with permission.)

presumed low specificity of athlete's ECG. In the authors' experience, among 42,386 athletes initially screened by history, physical examination, and 12-lead ECG, 3,914 (9%) were referred for further examination, and 879 (2%) were ultimately disqualified for cardiovascular reasons [29]. Therefore, the percentage of false positive results (ie, athletes with a normal heart but positive screening findings) requiring additional testing, mainly echocardiography, was only 7%, with a modest proportional impact on cost.

Summary

In conclusion, the Italian screening protocol essentially based on ECG—which has been used for preparticipation evaluation of millions of Italian athletes over a 25-year period—has adequate sensitivity and specificity for detection of potentially dangerous cardiovascular diseases, and substantially reduces mortality of young competitive athletes, mostly by preventing SCD from cardiomyopathy [5,6,29]. The results of the Italian preparticipation evaluation program have significant implications for implementing worldwide this screening strategy for prevention of athletic field sudden death.

References

[1] Maron BJ. Sudden death in young athletes. N Engl J Med 2003;349:1064–75.
[2] Corrado D, Basso C, Thiene G. Assay: sudden death in young athletes. Lancet 2005;366(Suppl 1):S47–8.
[3] Maron BJ, Roberts WC, McAllister MA, et al. Sudden death in young athletes. Circulation 1980;62:218–29.
[4] Corrado D, Thiene G, Nava A, et al. Sudden death in young competitive athletes: clinico-pathologic correlations in 22 cases. Am J Med 1990;89:588–96.
[5] Corrado D, Basso C, Schiavon M, et al. Screening for hypertrophic cardiomyopathy in young athletes. N Engl J Med 1998;339:364–9.
[6] Corrado D, Pelliccia A, Bjørnstad HH, et al. Cardiovascular preparticipation screening of young competitive athletes for prevention of sudden death: proposal for a common European protocol. Consensus statement of the Study Group of Sport Cardiology of the Working Group of Cardiac Rehabilitation and Exercise Physiology and the Working Group of Myocardial and Pericardial Diseases of the European Society of Cardiology. Eur Heart J 2005;26:516–24.
[7] Maron BJ, Thompson PD, Ackerman MJ, et al. American Heart Association Council on Nutrition, Physical Activity, and Metabolism. Recommendations and considerations related to preparticipation screening for cardiovascular abnormalities in competitive athletes: 2007 update: a scientific statement from the American Heart Association Council on

Nutrition, Physical Activity, and Metabolism: endorsed by the American College of Cardiology Foundation. Circulation 2007;115:1643–55.

[8] Thompson PD, Franklin BA, Balady GJ, et al. American Heart Association Council on Nutrition, Physical Activity, and Metabolism; American Heart Association Council on Clinical Cardiology; American College of Sports Medicine. Exercise and acute cardiovascular events placing the risks into perspective: a scientific statement from the American Heart Association Council on Nutrition, Physical Activity, and Metabolism and the Council on Clinical Cardiology. Circulation 2007;115:2358–68.

[9] Van Camp SP, Bloor CM, Mueller FO, et al. Nontraumatic sports death in high school and college athletes. Med Sci Sports Exerc 1995;27:641–7.

[10] Corrado D, Basso C, Rizzoli G, et al. Does sports activity enhance the risk of sudden death in adolescents and young adults? J Am Coll Cardiol 2003;42: 1959–63.

[11] Maron BJ, Shirani J, Poliac LC, et al. Sudden death in young competitive athletes. Clinical, demographics, and pathological profiles. JAMA 1996;276: 199–204.

[12] Thiene G, Nava A, Corrado D, et al. Right ventricular cardiomyopathy and sudden death in young people. N Engl J Med 1988;318:129–33.

[13] Maron BJ, Chaitman BR, Ackerman MJ, et al. Working Groups of the American Heart Association Committee on Exercise, Cardiac Rehabilitation, and Prevention; Councils on Clinical Cardiology and Cardiovascular Disease in the Young. Recommendations for physical activity and recreational sports participation for young patients with genetic cardiovascular diseases. Circulation 2004;109:2807–16.

[14] Corrado D, Basso C, Schiavon M, Maron BJ, Thiene G. Preparticipation screening strategies for prevention of sudden death in young competitive athletes: 12-lead ECG makes the difference. Heart Rhythm 2005;2:S80.

[15] Corrado D, McKenna WJ. Appropriate interpretation of athlete's electrocardiogram saves lives as well as money. Eur Heart J 2007;28:1920–2.

[16] Ryan MP, Cleland JGF, French JA, et al. The standard electrocardiogram as a screening test for hypertrophic cardiomyopathy. Am J Cardiol 1995;76: 689–94.

[17] Melacini P, Fasoli G, Canciani B, et al. Hypertrophic cardiomyopathy: Two-dimensional echocardiografic score versus clinical and electrocardiographic findings. Clin Cardiol 1989;12:443–52.

[18] Foote CB, Michaud GF. The Athlete's electrocardiogram: distinguishing normal from abnormal. In:

Estes NAM, Salem DN, Wang PJ, editors. Sudden cardiac death in the athlete. Armonk (NY): Futura Publishing; 1998. p. 101–13.

[19] Pelliccia A, Maron BJ, Culasso F, et al. Clinical significance of abnormal electrocardiographic patterns in trained athletes. Circulation 2000;102:278–84.

[20] Sharma S, Whyte G, Elliott P, et al. Electrocardiographic changes in 1000 highly trained junior elite athletes. Br J Sports Med 1999;33:319–24.

[21] Somauroo JD, Pyatt JR, Jackson M, et al. An echocardiographic assessment of cardiac morphology and common ECG findings in teenage professional soccer players: reference ranges for use in screening. Heart 2001;85:649–54.

[22] Douglas PS, O'Toole ML, Hiller WDB, et al. Electrocardiographic diagnosis of exercise-induced left ventricular hypertrophy. Am Heart J 1988;116: 784–90.

[23] Pelliccia F, Cianfrocca C, Cristofani R, et al. Electrocardiographic findings in patients with hypertrophic cardiomyopathy. Relation to presenting features and prognosis. J Electrocardiol 1990;23: 213–22.

[24] Marcus FI. Prevalence of T-wave inversion beyond V1 in young normal individuals and usefulness for the diagnosis of arrhythmogenic right ventricular cardiomyopathy/dysplasia. Am J Cardiol 2005;95: 1070–1.

[25] Pelliccia A, Culasso F, Di Paolo F, et al. Prevalence of abnormal electrocardiograms in a large, unselected athletic population undergoing preparticipation cardiovascular screening. Eur Heart J 2007;28: 2006–10.

[26] Corrado D, Michieli P, Schiavon M, et al. Prevalence and clinical significance of right precordial T-wave inversion at electrocardiographic preparticipation screening: a prospective study on 3086 young competitive athletes [abstract]. Circulation 2007; in press.

[27] McKenna WJ, Spirito P, Desnos M, et al. Experience from clinical genetics in hypertrophic cardiomyopathy: proposal for new diagnostic criteria in adult members of affected families. Heart 1997;77: 130–2.

[28] Pelliccia A, Di Paolo FM, Corrado D, et al. Evidence for efficacy of the Italian national pre-participation screening programme for identification of hypertrophic cardiomyopathy in competitive athletes. Eur Heart J 2006;27:2196–200.

[29] Corrado D, Basso C, Pavei A, et al. Trends in sudden cardiovascular death in young competitive athletes after implementation of a preparticipation screening program. JAMA 2006;296:1593–601.

Hypertrophic Cardiomyopathy and Other Causes of Sudden Cardiac Death in Young Competitive Athletes, with Considerations for Preparticipation Screening and Criteria for Disqualification

Barry J. Maron, MD

Hypertrophic Cardiomyopathy Center, Minneapolis Heart Institute Foundation, 920 E. 28th Street, Suite 60, Minneapolis, MN 55407, USA

The highly conditioned young competitive athlete projects the imagery of the healthiest facet of our society [1]. Nevertheless, youthful athletes may die suddenly, often during sports competition or training [2–13]. Such catastrophes are always unexpected events and while relatively uncommon, nevertheless achieve high visibility and convey a particularly tragic and devastating impact upon the medical and lay communities. The fact that many such athletes may have performed at exceptionally high levels of excellence for long periods of time with severe cardiovascular malformations has long intrigued investigators and the lay public.

Although initially reported and promoted in the United States in the early 1980s [13], over the past several years interest and concern have heightened considerably regarding the causes of sudden and unexpected deaths in young trained athletes [6]. Once regarded as rare personal and family tragedies, these deaths have been increasingly integrated into the public discourse. Consequently, the underlying cardiovascular causes have been the focus of several reports from the United States and Europe, and a large measure of clarification has resulted [1–13]. Indeed, the risks associated with participation in organized competitive sports are diverse, and range from sudden collapse from a variety of underlying (and usually unsuspected) cardiovascular diseases

[1–13] to nonpenetrating, chest impact-related catastrophes [14,15]. Recognition that athletic field deaths are often caused by detectable cardiovascular lesions has also stimulated substantial interest, in both in the United States and Europe, in the preparticipation screening process in high school and college-aged athletes [16,17], as well as in issues related to the criteria for eligibility and disqualification from competitive sports [18,19].

Cardiovascular causes of sudden death in young athletes

A competitive athlete is defined as one who participates in an organized team or individual sport which requires regular competition against others as a central component, places a high premium on excellence and achievement, and requires vigorous and intense training in a systematic fashion [18]. This definition is arbitrary, and it should be underscored that many individuals participate in recreational sports in a truly competitive fashion.

Several autopsy-based studies have documented the cardiovascular diseases responsible for sudden death in young competitive athletes [2–13]. These structural abnormalities are independent of the normal physiologic adaptations in cardiac dimensions evident in many trained athletes, usually consisting of increased left ventricular (LV) end-diastolic cavity dimension and mass, and occasionally LV wall thickness [12,20–22]. It is important to recognize that assignment

E-mail address: hcm.maron@mhif.org

of strict prevalence figures for the relative occurrence of various cardiovascular diseases in studies of sudden death in athletes are unavoidably influenced by selection biases and other limitations in the absence of systematic national or international registries.

Nevertheless, even with these considerations in mind, it has been convincingly demonstrated that the vast majority of sudden deaths in young athletes (those under age 35) are due to a diverse array of primarily congenital cardiovascular diseases (about 15) (Fig. 1) [2,7,8]. Indeed, virtually any disease capable of causing sudden death in young people may potentially do so in young competitive athletes. While these diseases may be relatively common in young athletes dying suddenly, each is distinctly uncommon within the general population.

Hypertrophic cardiomyopathy

The single most common cardiovascular cause of sudden death in young athletes in the United States,

and the focal point of this article, is hypertrophic cardiomyopathy (HCM) [2,6,7,10,23,24], accounting for about 35% of such events (Figs. 1–3). Indeed, the three most recent (and highly visible) sudden deaths or cardiac arrests occurring among United States professional athletes were each due to HCM (Jason Collier, Thomas Herrion, and Jiri Fischer in basketball, football, and hockey, respectively), as well as one other notable sudden death in a Cameroon soccer player (with previously diagnosed HCM) occurring during a televised international match [12].

HCM is a primary and familial cardiac malformation with heterogeneous clinical and morphologic expression, complex pathophysiology, and diverse clinical course. It is the most common genetic cardiovascular malformation occurring in about 1 in 500 of the general population [25]. Eleven mutated sarcomeric genes have been associated with HCM, most commonly beta-myosin heavy chain (the first identified) and myosin-binding protein C [24,26]. Nine other genes appear to

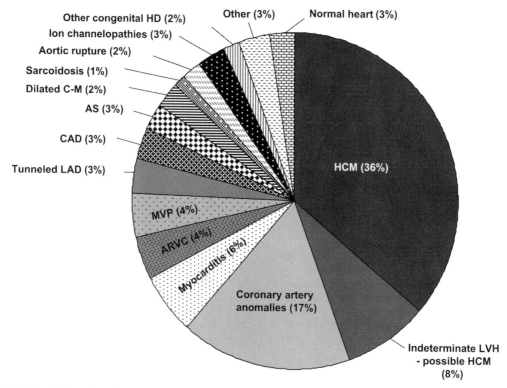

Fig. 1. Distribution of cardiovascular causes of sudden death in 1,435 young competitive athletes. ARVC, arrhythmogenic right ventricular cardiomyopathy; AS, aortic stenosis; CAD, coronary artery disease; C-M, cardiomyopathy; HCM, hypertrophic cardiomyopathy; HD, heart disease; LAD, left anterior descending; LVH, left ventricular hypertrophy. (*Courtesy of* the Minneapolis Heart Institute Registry, 1980–2005, Minneapolis, MN; with permission.)

account for far fewer cases and include troponin T and I, α-tropomyosin, regulatory and essential myosin light chains, titin, α-actin, α-myosin heavy chain, and muscle LIM protein (MLP). This intergene diversity is compounded by considerable intragenetic heterogeneity, with multiple different mutations identified in each gene (total n = more than 400 individual mutations) (http://cardiogenomics.med.harvard.edu). Characteristic diversity of the HCM phenotype, even within closely related family members, is likely attributable to both the disease –causing mutations and the influence of modifier genes and environmental factors. Neither the complete number of genes nor HCM-causing mutations are known, and many others undoubtedly remain to be identified.

In addition, nonsarcomeric protein mutations in two genes involved in cardiac metabolism (eg, gamma-2-regulatory subunit of the AMP-activated protein kinase [PRKAG2] and lysosome-associated membrane protein 2 [LAMP-2; Danon disease]) are responsible for primary cardiac glycogen storage cardiomyopathies in older children and young adults [27]. The clinical presentations mimic or are indistinguishable from sarcomeric HCM, but are often associated with ventricular pre-excitation [27].

Sudden death in HCM is most common in children and young adults (under age 30), usually in individuals who previously have been asymptomatic (or only mildly symptomatic) [23,24,28]. Therefore, such catastrophes usually occur without warning signs and are often the first clinical manifestation of the disease, caused by primary ventricular tachycardia/fibrillation (Fig. 4). Although most HCM patients die while sedentary or during mild exertion, a substantial proportion collapse during or just after vigorous physical activity [8,12]. The latter observation, as well as evidence that HCM is the most common cause of sudden death in young competitive athletes [2,5–8,10,12] and that athletes with HCM (and other cardiac diseases) usually collapse during training or competition [2], support the view that intense physical activity can represent a trigger for sudden death. Therefore, it follows that recommending disqualification of athletes with HCM from intense competitive sports is a prudent management strategy [18,19]. The one sport which provides the most practical alternative to disqualification is competitive golf, which is permitted under consensus panel guidelines [18].

Clinical diagnosis of HCM is generally based on the definition (by two-dimensional echocardiography) of the most characteristic morphologic feature of the disease: that is, asymmetric thickening of the LV wall associated with a non-dilated cavity, and in the absence of another cardiac or systemic disease capable of producing the magnitude of hypertrophy evident (eg, systemic hypertension or aortic stenosis) [2,24,29] (see Figs. 2 and 3). Because outflow obstruction is uncommon under resting conditions [24,28], the well-described clinical features of dynamic obstruction to left ventricular outflow, such as a loud systolic ejection murmur, marked systolic anterior motion (SAM) of the mitral valve, or partial premature closure of the aortic valve, are not required for the diagnosis of HCM. However, it is now evident that a substantial proportion of patients without obstruction at rest develop outflow tract gradients caused by SAM with physiologic exercise [30].

Based on both echocardiographic and necropsy studies in large numbers of patients, it is apparent that the HCM disease spectrum is characterized by vast structural diversity with regard to the patterns and extent of LV hypertrophy [31–33] (see Fig. 3). Indeed, virtually all possible patterns of wall thickening occur in HCM, and no single phenotypic expression can be considered classic or typical of this disease. While many patients show diffusely distributed hypertrophy, fully 30% have wall thickening confined to only one segment of the LV. Average absolute LV thickness reported from tertiary center cohorts is 21 mm to 22 mm [23,31].

Wall thickness is profoundly increased in many patients, including some showing the most severe hypertrophy observed in any cardiac disease, with 60 mm the most extreme dimension reported to date [33]. Extreme hypertrophy (maximum wall thickness greater than or equal to 30 mm) is, in fact, regarded as an independent risk factor for sudden death in young HCM patients [34]. On the other hand, the HCM phenotype is not invariably expressed as a greatly thickened left ventricle, as in some genetically affected individuals showing only a mild increase of 13 mm to 15 mm, or even normal wall thicknesses (less than or equal to 12 mm), usually in asymptomatic family members identified by virtue of pedigree studies [35]. Therefore, no specific absolute LV wall thickness is inconsistent with the diagnosis of HCM [24,31,36].

In some young athletes with segmental hypertrophy confined to the anterior ventricular septum (eg, wall thicknesses, 13 mm–15 mm), it may be difficult to distinguish mild morphologic expression of HCM from extreme manifestations of physiologic LV hypertrophy, which represents adaptation to athletic training (ie, athlete's heart) [12,35]. In trained athletes within this morphologic "gray zone" of overlap (about 2% of elite male athletes) [21], the differential diagnosis and ambiguity between physiologic athlete's heart and HCM (without outflow obstruction) can often be resolved by clinical assessment and noninvasive testing (Fig. 5) [12,35]. This diagnostic

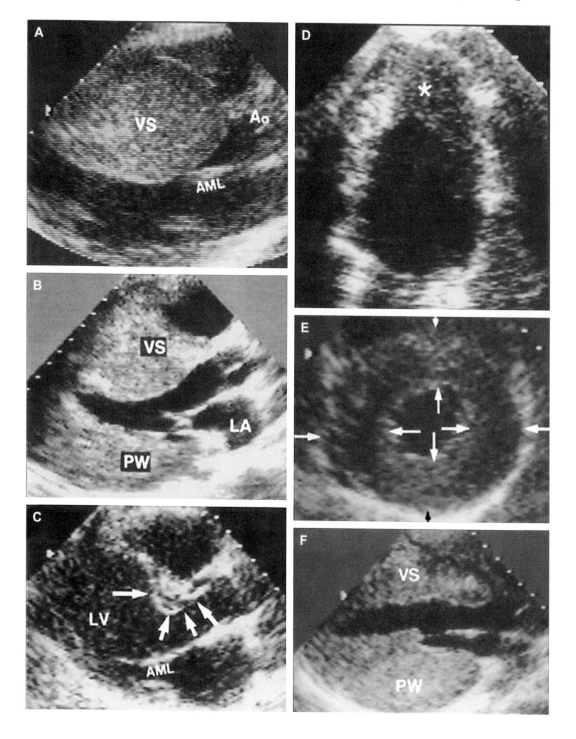

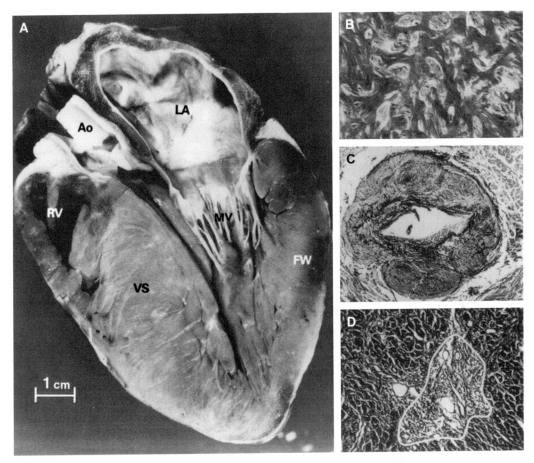

Fig. 3. Morphologic components of disease process in HCM. (*A*) Heart sectioned in cross-sectional long-axis plane. LV wall thickening is asymmetric, confined primarily to the ventricular septum (VS), which bulges prominently into small LV outflow tract. FW, left ventricular free wall; Ao, aorta; LA, left atrium; RV, right ventricle; (*B*) Septal myocardium shows greatly disorganized architecture with adjacent hypertrophied cardiac muscle cells arranged perpendicularly and obliquely; (*C*) Intramural coronary artery with thickened wall, due primarily to medial hypertrophy, and narrowed lumen; (*D*) Demarcated area of replacement fibrosis in septum. (*From* Maron BJ. Hypertrophic cardiomyopathy. Lancet 1997;350:127–33; with permission.)

strategy involves the application of a number of noninvasive parameters, such as reduced LV mass with short deconditioning periods (best assessed with serial MRI) or LV end-diastolic dimension greater than 55 mm, both of which favor physiologic athlete's heart [12,35]. Conversely, an HCM diagnosis would be most likely with abnormal Doppler-derived LV diastolic

Fig. 2. Heterogeneous pattern and extent of left ventricular wall thickening in HCM. Echocardiographic images in enddiastole. (*A*) Massive asymmetric hypertrophy of ventricular septum (VS) with thickness >50 mm; (*B*) Septal hypertrophy with distal portion considerably thicker than proximal region; (*C*) Hypertrophy confined to proximal septum just below aortic valve (*arrows*); (*D*) Hypertrophy localized to LV apex (*) (ie, apical HCM); (*E*) Relatively mild hypertrophy in concentric (symmetric) pattern showing similar or identical thicknesses within each segment (paired arrows); (*F*) Inverted pattern with posterior free wall (PW) thicker (40 mm) than anterior VS Calibration marks = 1 cm. Ao, aorta; AML, anterior mitral leaflet; LA, left atrium. (*From* Klues HG, Schiffers A, Maron BJ. Phenotypic spectrum and patterns of left ventricular hypertrophy in hypertrophic cardiomyopathy: morphologic observations and significance as assessed by two-dimensional echocardiography in 600 patients. J Am Coll Cardiol 1995;26:1699–708; reproduced with the permission of American College of Cardiology.)

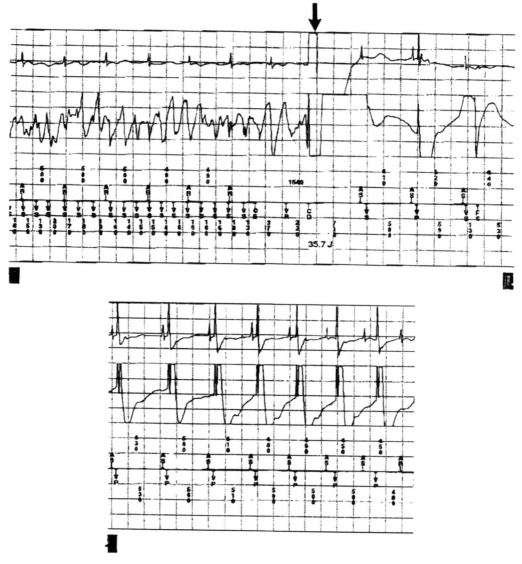

Fig. 4. Mechanism of sudden death in HCM. Demonstrated by a stored intracardiac ventricular electrogram from a 28-year-old asymptomatic patient with extreme LV hypertrophy (ventricular septal thickness, 36 mm) as the sole risk factor. Patient who received an implantable cardioverter-defibrillator for primary prevention of sudden death. Spontaneous onset of ventricular fibrillation is automatically sensed and terminated by a defibrillation shock (*arrow*), immediately restoring sinus rhythm.

filling or relaxation indices, a family member with HCM, or small LV cavity in diastole (less than 45 mm). MRI also has potential value for resolving the HCM versus athlete's heart dilemma in selected athletes by virtue of its superiority over echocardiography in identifying segmental hypertrophy in the anterolateral LV free wall or at the apex (Fig. 6) [32].

Commercial laboratory genetic testing

Commercial laboratory testing is now available in HCM, with the potential for achieving an unequivocal DNA-based diagnosis in athlete's heart versus HCM or other clinical scenarios (http://www.hpcgg.org/LMM/tests.html). If a proband is positive for one of the 10 most common HCM-causing mutant genes tested in the panel,

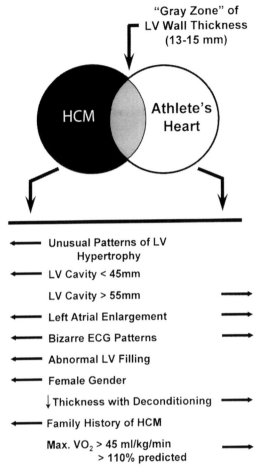

Fig. 5. Chart showing criteria used to distinguish HCM from athlete's heart when the LV wall thickness is within the shaded gray zone of overlap (13 mm–15 mm), consistent with both diagnoses. This is assumed to be the nonobstructive form of HCM in this article, as the presence of substantial mitral valve systolic anterior motion would, per se, confirm the diagnosis of HCM in an athlete. HCM may involve a variety of abnormalities, including heterogeneous distribution of left ventricular hypertrophy (LVH) in which asymmetry is prominent, and adjacent regions may be of greatly different thicknesses, with sharp transitions evident between segments; also, patterns in which the anterior ventricular septum is spared from the hypertrophic process and the region of predominant thickening may be in the posterior portion of septum or anterolateral or posterior free wall or apex. ↓, decreased; LA, left atrial. (*From* Maron BJ, Pelliccia A, Spirito P. Cardiac disease in young trained athletes: Insights into methods for distinguishing athlete's heart from structural heart disease with particular emphasis on hypertrophic cardiomyopathy. Circulation 1995; 91:1596–601; reproduced with permission of American Heart Association.)

the test result is definitive. On the other hand, such genetic testing has potential limitations. For example, negative tests in probands while common, are nondiagnostic because they may frequently represent false negative results. In addition, commercial testing is costly (in the range of $5,000 for all 10 genes), and it is presently unpredictable as to whether that expense will always be covered by insurance carriers. However, if the gene defect responsible for HCM in the family becomes known, then other family members can easily be tested definitively and inexpensively.

Congenital coronary artery anomalies

Second in importance and frequency to HCM is a variety of congenital malformations of the coronary arteries, the most common of which is anomalous origin of the left main coronary artery from the right (anterior) sinus of Valsalva (see Fig. 1) [2,37,38]. These anomalies require a high index of clinical suspicion [39], given the characteristic absence of ECG and stress test abnormalities [38].

Young individuals with anomalous left main coronary artery may die suddenly as the first manifestation of their disease, although a minority experience angina, syncope, or even acute myocardial infarction. The vast majority of these events are related to exertion. Indeed, occurrence of one or more episodes of exertional syncope in a young athlete necessitates exclusion of this coronary anomaly. In youthful athletes it may be possible to identify (or raise strong suspicion of) anomalous left main (or right) coronary artery using cross-sectional two-dimensional or transesophageal echocardiography or CT angiogram [39,40], which can then lead to definitive confirmation with coronary arteriography or CT angiogram. These clinical considerations are of particular importance because coronary malformations are amenable to corrective surgery.

Other unusual variants of coronary arterial anatomy have been reported rarely as causes of exercise-related sudden deaths in young athletic individuals [2,37]. These include hypoplasia of some portion of the coronary circulation, left anterior descending or right coronary artery emanating from the pulmonary trunk, or coronary arterial intersusception occlusion of the coronary lumen.

Arrhythmogenic right ventricular cardiomyopathy

This is a familial condition, which may be associated with important ventricular or supraventricular arrhythmias, and is a cause of sudden death

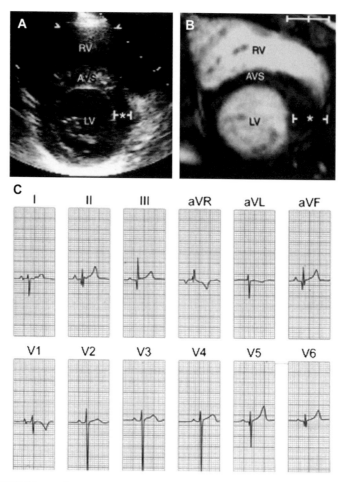

Fig. 6. Diagnosis of HCM by cardiac magnetic resonance (CMR) imaging. Studies from a 13-year-old identical twin with nonobstructive HCM. Two-dimensional stop-frame echocardiogram (*A*) and comparative CMR imaging (*B*) images acquired in the short-axis plane in end-diastole at mitral valve level; and 12-lead ECG (*C*). (*A*) Echocardiogram shows normal thickness in all LV wall segments, including anterior ventricular septum (AVS) and the contiguous portion of anterolateral free wall (*). Stop-frame image is representative of all cross-sectional images obtained in this patient. (*B*) CMR image showing segmental area of hypertrophy confined to the anterolateral LV free wall (20 mm) and a small portion of the contiguous AVS (*), which was identified only with CMR. Shown in the same cross-sectional plane as the echocardiogram shown in (*A*); RV, right ventricle. (*C*) Distinctly abnormal ECG showing Q waves in inferior leads II, III and AVF, and V6, deep S-waves in right precordial leads, and diminished precordial R-waves. Recorded at full standard, 1 mV = 10 mm. AVS, anterior ventricular septum; RV, right ventricle. Calibration marks in (*A*) and (*B*) are 1 cm apart; magnification of images in the two panels is not identical. (*From* Rickers C, Wilke NM, Jerosch-Herold M, et al. Utility of cardiac magnetic resonance imaging in the diagnosis of hypertrophic cardiomyopathy. Circulation 2005;112:855–61; reproduced with permission of American Heart Association.)

in the young (see Fig. 1) [41–45]. Arrhythmogenic right ventricular cardiomyopathy (ARVC) is characterized morphologically by myocyte death, with replacement by fibrous and/or adipose tissue in the right ventricle (see Fig. 6). This disease process may be segmental or diffusely involve the right ventricle.

Italian investigators have persistently reported ARVC to be the most common cause of sudden death in young competitive athletes in the Veneto region of northeastern Italy. While ARVC is also a component of the United States experience with athletic field deaths, its frequency is in the range of less than 5% [2,5,6,8]. The explanation for such differences is uncertain, although it is possible that the relatively frequent occurrence of ARVC in Italy reflects a unique genetic substrate [41–45]. Paradoxically, the low frequency with which

HCM is apparently responsible for sudden death in Italian competitive athletes is likely due to the long-standing 25-year systematic national program for the cardiovascular assessment of competitive athletes [11,17,46]. This Italian screening effort has apparently identified and disqualified disproportionate numbers of trained athletes with HCM, because of the fact that it is more easily identifiable clinically than is ARVC [47].

Less common causes of sudden death in young athletes (accounting for 3%–8%) include myocarditis, dilated cardiomyopathy, aortic dissection and rupture (usually caused by Marfan syndrome), sarcoidosis, valvular heart disease (eg, mitral valve prolapse or aortic valve stenosis), and atherosclerotic coronary artery disease (see Fig. 1) [2,5–8]. Also, a small number of athletes die suddenly without evidence of structural cardiovascular disease, even after careful gross and histologic examination of the heart. In such instances (about 2% of our series), it may not be possible to definitively exclude noncardiac factors (eg, drug abuse) as responsible for the death, or to know whether careful inspection of the specialized conducting system and associated vasculature with serial sectioning (no longer standard part of the medical examiners' protocol) would have revealed clinically relevant abnormalities [48]. Given the absence of a clinical cardiovascular evaluation, one can only speculate on the potential etiologies of many such deaths. However, it is likely that some are caused by previously unidentified Wolff-Parkinson-White syndrome, ion channelopathies such as long QT or Brugada syndromes, and catecholaminergic polymorphic ventricular tachycardia, or possibly, undetected segmental ARVC or subtle morphologic forms of HCM.

In about 5% of United States athletic field deaths, a segment of left anterior descending coronary artery was tunneled (ie, surrounded by myocardium for 1 cm–3 cm) in the absence of another structural anomaly [2,5–8]. It has been suggested that such short "tunneled" segments of major coronary arteries (ie, myocardial "bridges") constitute a potentially lethal anatomic variant which may cause sudden unexpected death in susceptible, but otherwise healthy young individuals during exertion [49].

Sudden unexpected death, nonfatal stroke, and acute myocardial infarction in trained athletes have been attributed to illicit substance abuse with cocaine, anabolic steroids, or dietary and nutritional supplements [12,50–52]; the latter are often consumed to enhance sports performance or mask other drugs during surveillance. Popular supplements for promoting athletic performance are compounds such as *ma huang*, an herbal source of ephedrine (ie, elemental ephedra) and a cardiac stimulant which is potentially arrhythmogenic [6,52]. Causal linkage between dietary supplements and cardiovascular events in otherwise healthy people is largely by inference, based on the close temporal relation between ingestion of the compound and adverse consequences [52].

Commotio cordis

Blows to the chest, and specifically the precordium, can trigger ventricular fibrillation without structural injury to ribs, sternum, or heart itself (commotio cordis) [14,15,53]. Indeed, these events are more common causes of athletic field deaths than many of the aforementioned specific cardiovascular diseases. Commotio cordis is frequently caused by projectiles which are implements of the game, and strike the chest at a broad range of velocities. For example, hockey pucks or lacrosse balls, which may strike up to 90 mph, but more frequently with only modest force (eg, a pitched baseball striking a young batter at 30 mph–40 mph), and with smaller impact areas [54]. Commotio cordis may also occur by virtue of bodily contact, such as a karate blow or when outfielders collide while tracking a baseball.

Based on clinical observations and an experimental animal model (which closely replicates commotio cordis), the mechanism by which ventricular fibrillation and sudden death occurs requires a blow directly over the heart, exquisitely timed to within a narrow 10-ms to 30-ms window just before the T-wave peak during the vulnerable phase of repolarization [53]. Basic electrophysiologic mechanisms of commotio cordis are largely unresolved, although selective mechanical activation of the ion channels appears to play a role [55,56].

Only about 15% of commotio cordis victims survive, usually associated with timely cardiopulmonary resuscitation and defibrillation [12,15]. There are reports of both successful and unsuccessful resuscitation with automated external defibrillators [12]. Strategies for primary prevention of commotio cordis include innovations in sports equipment design. While softer-than-normal ("safety") baseballs reduce the frequency of ventricular fibrillation under experimental conditions [53], such implements do not provide absolute protection on the athletic field [15]. Chest barriers with proven efficacy in preventing commotio cordis are not yet available and, under experimental conditions, commercially available chest protectors have proven ineffective in preventing ventricular fibrillation [57].

Prevalence and significance of the problem

Sudden unexpected death caused by cardiovascular disease during competitive sports is rare in high school students participating in organized interscholastic sports (ie, about 1 in 200,000 participants per year or 1 in 60,000 participants over a 3-year high school period) [58]. Somewhat lower estimates for the risk of sudden death have been reported for adult joggers or marathon road racing runners [57,59,60]. The automated external defibrillator has proven effective in reducing sudden death on the running course [60]. Preliminary data from a 26-year national registry on sudden death in athletes showed that such events in competitive athletes in the United States number about 125 each year, 5- to 10-fold more common than previously estimated [8]. Extrapolation of these data suggest that one young athlete dies suddenly every 3 days, and that one such athlete with HCM dies every 2 weeks.

The emotional and social impact of athletic field catastrophes remains high. The competitive athlete symbolizes the healthiest segment of our society and the unexpected collapse of such young people is a powerful event that inevitably strikes to the core sensibilities of both the lay public and physician community [1]. For these reasons, sudden death in young athletes will continue to represent an important medical issue and public health problem. Indeed, it is the responsibility of the medical community to create a fully informed public and to pursue early detection of the causes of catastrophic events in young athletes where prudent and practical. On the other hand, because such events are particularly uncommon with respect to the vast numbers of athletes participating safely in sports, it is important that information about athletic field deaths should not create undo anxiety among young athletes and their families.

Demographics

Based primarily on data assembled from broad-based United States populations [2,6–8], a profile of young competitive athletes who die suddenly has emerged. Such athletes participate in a large number and variety of sports, with the most common basketball and football (about 60%), probably reflecting the high participation level in these popular team sports as well as the physical intensity required. In Europe, soccer is most frequently associated with sudden death in athletes.

The vast majority of athletic field deaths occur in men (about 90%). This relative infrequency in women probably reflects lower participation rates, sometimes less intense levels of training, and the fact that women do not engage in some of the higher-risk sports (eg, football). Most athletes are involved in high school sports at the time of death (about 75%), and less commonly in college or professional competition.

The vast majority of athletes who die suddenly with HCM or other underlying diseases are free of symptoms or suspicion of cardiovascular disease. Sudden collapse usually occurs with physical exertion, predominantly in the late afternoon and early evening hours, corresponding to the peak periods of competition and training, and particularly in organized team sports, such as football and basketball [2,6]. In addition, underlying genetic heart diseases are more likely to cause sudden unexpected death in trained athletes than in their sedentary counterparts [43]. These observations substantiate that, in the presence of cardiovascular disease, physical activity represents a trigger and important precipitating factor for sudden death in athletes.

Although the majority of sudden deaths in competitive athletes have been reported in white males, a substantial proportion (more than 40%) are African-Americans [7], including the majority of HCM-related athletic field deaths (Fig. 7) [2]. The substantial number of HCM sudden deaths in young black male athletes contrasts sharply with the infrequent identification of black patients with HCM in hospital-based populations. These observations emphasize the disproportionately lesser access to subspecialty medical care between the African-American and white communities in the United States, which makes it less likely that young black males will receive the diagnosis of HCM. Consequently, African-American athletes with HCM are also less likely to be disqualified from competition to reduce their risk for sudden death, in accordance with the recommendations of Bethesda Conference #36 [18].

Mechanisms and resuscitation

In the vast majority of athletes with HCM and other cardiac diseases, cardiac arrest results from electrical instability with primary ventricular

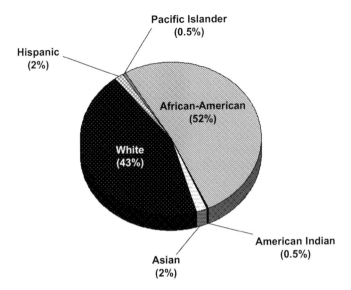

Fig. 7. Sudden death in young athletes due to HCM, with respect to race. Although HCM is very uncommonly diagnosed clinically in African-Americans, the majority of sudden deaths on the athletic field due to HCM are in young black males.

tachyarrhythmias (see Fig. 4). The major exception to this principle is Marfan syndrome, in which death is usually caused by aortic dissection and rupture. However, regardless of mechanism, only a minority of athletes with cardiovascular disease who collapse on the athletic field are successfully resuscitated. More widespread dissemination of automatic external defibrillators available for public access by nontraditional responders in schools and at athletic events would be expected to result in the survival of greater numbers of such athletes.

Screening and preparticipation detection of cardiovascular abnormalities

Detection of cardiovascular abnormalities with the potential for significant morbidity or sudden death is the important objective of the widespread practice of preparticipation screening of high school and college-aged athletes. There is a general consensus within a benevolent society that a responsibility exists on the part of physicians to initiate prudent efforts for the identification of life-threatening diseases in athletes, for the purpose of minimizing the cardiovascular risks associated with sports participation [16–19]. Indeed, identification of asymptomatic patients with genetic diseases, such as HCM, ARVC, and the ion channel diseases (long QT syndrome and

Brugada syndrome) has taken on much greater significance with the recent application of the implantable cardioverter-defibrillator for primary prevention of sudden death in high-risk individuals [61,62]. However, there is also a consensus that the return of athletes with potentially lethal cardiovascular disease to competition, based explicitly on the presence of an implantable defibrillator, is not advisable [18].

Major obstacles to any preparticipation screening program are the large reservoir of young competitive athletes eligible for evaluation (about 10–12 million in the United States), and the uncommon occurrence of the cardiovascular causes of sudden death within a young athlete population (estimated overall prevalence of 0.5% or less) [16]. Customary cardiovascular screening practice for United States high school and college athletes is confined to history and physical examination [16], a strategy that lacks sufficient power to identify certain important cardiovascular abnormalities consistently. For example, while the nonobstructive (at rest) form of HCM is the single most common disease entity to be targeted, its clinical recognition or suspicion raised by screening can be expected to occur relatively infrequently because potential diagnostic markers such as loud heart murmur, syncope, or family history of sudden death may often be absent. In a retrospective study, only 3% of trained athletes who died suddenly of HCM and other heart diseases were suspected by preparticipation screening (with history and physical examination) to have cardiovascular abnormalities, and none were disqualified from competition [2].

The quality of the cardiovascular screening process for United States high school and college athletes has come under critical scrutiny [63,64]. However, improvements in the design of approved history and physical examination questionnaires have been noted over the past decade [65]. Nevertheless, the degree to which these changes can translate to greater numbers of athletes identified with cardiovascular disease will be difficult (if not impossible) to determine systematically with any precision. Legislation in several states continues to mandate that health care workers with vastly different levels of training and expertise (including chiropractors at naturopathic clinics) perform preparticipation sports examinations, often conducted under suboptimal conditions [16,65]. National standardization of high school and college preparticipation medical examinations, incorporating American Heart Association (AHA) recommendations (Table 1) [16], would provide the most practical and effective strategy for achieving the goal of detecting athletes who unknowingly harbor clinically relevant cardiovascular abnormalities.

A unique circumstance has existed in Italy where, for the last 25 or more years, federal government legislation (Medical Protection of Athletic Activities Act) has mandated national preparticipation screening and medical clearance for all young athletes engaged in organized sports programs [17,46]. Annual sports medicine evaluations in Italy routinely include history and physical examination, as well as 12-lead ECG. Because the electrocardiogram is abnormal in up to 95% of HCM patients [66], this test permits identification of many athletes previously undiagnosed with that disease [47]. Italian investigators have attributed a decline in the rate of sudden cardiac death during competitive sports to the long-standing systematic preparticipation screening program in that country, which routinely includes a 12-lead ECG [11,17,47].

Specifically, they report an almost 90% decline in the annual incidence of sudden cardiovascular death in competitive athletes (a result largely due to reduced mortality from cardiomyopathy) for the Veneto region of northeastern Italy [11]. This change in the death rate occurred in parallel with progressive implementation of nationwide mass

Table 1

The 12-element AHA recommendations for preparticipation cardiovascular screening of competitive athletes

Medical history[a]

Personal history

1. Exertional chest pain or discomfort
2. Unexplained syncope or near-syncope[b]
3. Excessive exertional and unexplained dyspnea or fatigue, associated with exercise
4. Prior recognition of a heart murmur
5. Elevated systemic blood pressure

Family history

6. Premature death (sudden and unexpected, or otherwise) before age 50 due to heart disease, in one or more relatives
7. Disability from heart disease in a close relative less than 50 years old
8. Specific knowledge of certain cardiac conditions in family members: hypertrophic or dilated cardiomyopathy, long QT syndrome or other ion channelopathies, Marfan syndrome, or clinically important arrhythmias

Physical examination

9. Heart murmur[c]
10. Femoral pulses to exclude aortic coarctation
11. Physical stigmata of Marfan syndrome
12. Brachial artery blood pressure (sitting position)[d]

[a] Parental verification is recommended for high school and middle school athletes.

[b] Judged not to be neurocardiogenic (vasovagal); of particular concern when related to exertion.

[c] Auscultation should be performed in both supine and standing positions (or with Valsalva maneuver), in particular to identify murmurs of dynamic left ventricular outflow tract obstruction.

[d] Preferably, taken initially in both arms.

screening and the increasing identification of affected athletes who were then disqualified from competitive sports to lower their risk.

Obstacles to implementing obligatory government-sponsored national with electrocardiography or echocardiography screening in the United States are outlined in detail in the 2007 AHA consensus statement on preparticipation screening [16]. These factors include the particularly large athlete population to be screened, major cost-benefit considerations, recognition that it is not possible to achieve a zero-risk circumstance in competitive sports, and most importantly, the lack of pre-existent resources in the form of dedicated medical personnel (including physicians) available to perform the athlete examinations and interpret their ECGs [16]. In addition, large population preparticipation screening with noninvasive testing is limited by the expected large numbers of false-positive (ie, borderline) examinations. Furthermore, there is the possibility of false-negative tests in which subtle but important lesions go undetected, as when echocardiography is performed in the pre-hypertrophic phase of HCM (usually less than 14 years old) [67], or when coronary anomalies cannot be recognized [38].

Criteria for sports eligibility and disqualification

When a cardiovascular abnormality is identified in a competitive athlete several considerations arise: (1) level of risk for sudden death if participation in organized sports continues; (2) likelihood that risk would be reduced if systematic training and competition were terminated; and (3) criteria to formulate appropriate eligibility or disqualification decisions. Unfortunately, on occasion the medical disqualification decision-making process can become polarized, given the personal aspirations of the athlete versus the mandate of the physician to protect patients from circumstances which could provoke unacceptable risks [1–3,6].

It should be underscored that the risk associated with intense physical exertion for sports participants with cardiovascular abnormalities is difficult to quantify with any precision, given the extreme and unpredictable physiologic circumstances to which individual athletes may be exposed. Indeed, only some HCM-related sudden deaths are associated with intense physical activity [24], and not all trained athletes with this disease die suddenly during their competitive phase [68].

In this regard, the American College of Cardiology (ACC) 36th Bethesda Conference [18] and European Society of Cardiology (ESC) [19], offers expert consensus panel recommendations and clear benchmarks for clinical practice. Panel guidelines for athletic eligibility or disqualification are predicated on the premise that intense sports training and competition increases sudden death risk in susceptible athletes with most forms of heart disease, and that risk is likely to be reduced or minimized by temporary or permanent withdrawal from sports participation. Indeed, the unique pressures of organized athletics are restrictive and do not allow individuals to exert strict control over their level of exertion, or reliably discern when cardiac symptoms arise which make it prudent to withdraw from physical activity. The

United States appellate court decision in Knapp v. Northwestern [3] supports the use of national association medical guidelines (such as the Bethesda Conference) in making disqualification recommendations for athletes. Therefore, team physicians would be prudent to rely on Bethesda Conference #36 [18] in making difficult eligibility-disqualification decisions, because it will likely play an important role as precedent in resolving future medical-legal disputes.

Under the ACC-Bethesda Conference #36, young athletes with the unequivocal diagnosis of HCM are discouraged from competitive athletic participation, with the exception of low-intensity sports (eg, golf and bowling) [18]. Other acquired diseases that are potentially reversible (such as myocarditis) can justify temporary withdrawal from competition, followed by resumption of organized sports activity after reversal and resolution of the disease state.

The ESC consensus report [19] is modeled largely after the Bethesda Conference [18]. While the two guidelines are very similar, the European recommendations are in some instances more restrictive in advising disqualification for certain cardiac conditions, including HCM, but also long QT syndrome and Marfan syndrome.

However, decisions to withdraw athletes from sports because of heart disease may be confounded by complex societal considerations and can prove difficult to implement, particularly when elite careers in sports are involved [1,3]. Many such athletes are highly motivated to remain in the competitive arena, may not fully appreciate the implications of the relevant medical information, or are nevertheless willing to accept the risks while resisting prudent recommendations to withdraw. However, in contrast to Italy [46], national standards linked to mandatory disqualification are not part of the United States health care system.

Improper over-diagnosis of cardiac disease may lead to unnecessary disqualification from athletics, thereby depriving some individuals of the psychological and economic benefits of competitive sports. As a cautionary note, physician judgment in making these medical eligibility and disqualification decisions can be impaired insidiously by extrinsic pressures imposed by relatives, fans, alumni, coaching staff and administrators, and particularly when athletes participate in "shopping" for multiple medical opinions until one is secured supporting continued sports participation. A measure of responsibility for these complex situations is attributable to societal attitudes that often attach exaggerated importance and materialism to organized sports [1].

In the United States the relationship between sports medicine and the law is complex, and involves tenuous relationships between physicians, athlete-patients, teams, and institutions. Indeed, liability issues relevant to the management of competitive athletes with cardiovascular disease have become of increasing concern to the practicing medical community, given that several athlete deaths have triggered disputes in court holding physicians accountable for alleged grievances. An evolving United States medical-legal framework is clarifying the standard of care associated with this clinical practice, while upholding the wisdom of withholding selected student-athletes with cardiovascular abnormalities from access to athletic programs and intense competitive sports, in an effort to significantly reduce exposure to medically unacceptable risks [69].

> The time you won your town the race
> We chaired you through the market-place;
> Man and boy stood cheering by,
> And home we brought you shoulder high.
> To-day, the road all runners come,
> Shoulder-high we bring you home,
> And set you at your threshold down,
> Townsman of a stiller town.
>
> *By Alfred Edward Housman, 1895*
> *To An Athlete Dying Young*

References

[1] Maron BJ. Sudden death in young athletes: lessons from the hank gathers affair. N Engl J Med 1993; 329:55–7.

[2] Maron BJ, Shirani J, Poliac LC, et al. Sudden death in young competitive athletes: clinical, demographic and pathological profiles. JAMA 1996;276:199–204.

[3] Maron BJ, Mitten MJ, Quandt EK, et al. Competitive athletes with cardiovascular disease—the case of Nicholas Knapp. N Engl J Med 1998;339:1623–5.

[4] Maron BJ. Cardiovascular risks to young persons on the athletic field. Ann Intern Med 1998;129:379–86.

[5] Van Camp SP, Bloor CM, Mueller FO, et al. Nontraumatic sports death in high school and college athletes. Med Sci Sports Exerc 1995;27:641–7.

[6] Maron BJ. Sudden death in young athletes. N Engl J Med 2003;349:1064–75.

[7] Maron BJ, Carney KP, Lever HM, et al. Relationship of race to sudden cardiac death in competitive athletes with hypertrophic cardiomyopathy. J Am Coll Cardiol 2003;41:974–80.

[8] Maron BJ, Doerer JJ, Haas TS, et al. Profile and frequency of sudden deaths in 1,463 young competitive athletes: from a 25-year US national registry, 1980–2005. Circulation 2006;114(Suppl II): II-830.

[9] Maron BJ, Towbin JA, Thiene G, et al. Contemporary definitions and classification of the cardiomyopathies. An American Heart Association Scientific Statement from the Council and Outcomes Research and Functional Genomics and Translational Biology Interdisciplinary Working Groups; and Council on Epidemiology and Prevention. Circulation 2006; 113:1807–16.

[10] Maron BJ, Epstein SE, Roberts WC. Causes of sudden death in the competitive athlete. J Am Coll Cardiol 1986;7:204–14.

[11] Corrado D, Basso C, Pavei A, et al. Trends in sudden cardiovascular death in young competitive athletes after implementation of a preparticipation screening program. JAMA 2006;1593–601.

[12] Maron BJ, Pelliccia A. The heart of trained athletes: cardiac remodeling and the risks of sports including sudden death. Circulation 2006;114:1633–44.

[13] Maron BJ, Roberts WC, McAllister HA, et al. Sudden death in young athletes. Circulation 1980;62:218–29.

[14] Maron BJ, Poliac LV, Kaplan JA, et al. Blunt impact to the chest leading to sudden death from cardiac arrest during sports activities. N Engl J Med 1995;33:337–42.

[15] Maron BJ, Gohman TE, Kyle SB, et al. Clinical profile and spectrum of commotio cordis. JAMA 2002; 287:1142–6.

[16] Maron BJ, Thompson PD, Ackerman MJ, et al. Recommendations and considerations related to preparticipation screening for cardiovascular abnormalities in competitive athletes: 2007 update: a scientific statement from the American Heart Association Council on Nutrition, Physical Activity, and Metabolism. Circulation 2007;115:1643–55.

[17] Corrado D, Pelliccia A, Björnstad HH, et al. Cardiovascular preparticipation screening of young competitive athletes for prevention of sudden death: proposal for a common European protocol. Consensus Statement of the Study Group of Sport Cardiology of the Working Group of Myocardial and Pericardial Diseases of the European Society of Cardiology. Eur Heart J 2005;26:510–24.

[18] Maron BJ, Zipes DP. 36th Bethesda Conference: eligibility recommendations for competitive athletes with cardiovascular abnormalities. J Am Coll Cardiol 2005;45:1312–75.

[19] Pelliccia A, Fagard R, Björnstad HH, et al. A European Society of Cardiology consensus document: recommendations for competitive sports participation in athletes with cardiovascular disease. Eur Heart J 2005;26:1422–45.

[20] Maron BJ. Structural features of the athlete heart as defined by echocardiography. J Am Coll Cardiol 1986;7:190–203.

[21] Pelliccia A, Maron BJ, Spataro A, et al. The upper limit of physiologic cardiac hypertrophy in highly trained elite athletes. N Engl J Med 1991;324:295–301.

[22] Pelliccia A, Maron BJ, Culasso F, et al. Athlete's heart in women: echocardiographic characterization of highly trained elite female athletes. JAMA 1996; 276:211–5.

[23] Maron BJ. Hypertrophic cardiomyopathy: a systematic review. JAMA 2002;287:1308–20.

[24] Maron BJ, McKenna WJ, Danielson GK, et al. American College of Cardiology/European Society of Cardiology clinical expert consensus document on hypertrophic cardiomyopathy. A report of the American College of Cardiology Task Force on Clinical Expert Consensus Documents and the European Society of Cardiology Committee for Practice Guidelines Committee to Develop an Expert Consensus Document on Hypertrophic Cardiomyopathy. J Am Coll Cardiol 2003;42: 1687–713.

[25] Maron BJ, Gardin JM, Flack JM, et al. Assessment of the prevalence of hypertrophic cardiomyopathy in a general population of young adults: echocardiographic analysis of 4111 subjects in the CARDIA Study. Circulation 1995;92:785–9.

[26] Seidman JG, Seidman CE. The genetic basis for cardiomyopathy: from mutation identification to mechanistic paradigms. Cell 2001;104:557–67.

[27] Arad M, Maron BJ, Gorham JM, et al. Glycogen storage diseases presenting as hypertrophic cardiomyopathy. N Engl J Med 2005;352:362–72.

[28] Spirito P, Seidman CE, McKenna WJ, et al. The management of hypertrophic cardiomyopathy. N Engl J Med 1997;336:775–85.

[29] Maron BJ, Epstein SE. Hypertrophic cardiomyopathy: a discussion of nomenclature. Am J Cardiol 1979;43:1242–4.

[30] Maron MS, Olivotto I, Zenovich AG, et al. Hypertrophic cardiomyopathy is predominantly a disease of left ventricular outflow tract obstruction. Circulation 2006;114:2232–9.

[31] Klues HG, Schiffers A, Maron BJ. Phenotypic spectrum and patterns of left ventricular hypertrophy in hypertrophic cardiomyopathy: morphologic observations and significance as assessed by two-dimensional echocardiography in 600 patients. J Am Coll Cardiol 1995;26:1699–708.

[32] Rickers C, Wilke NM, Jerosch-Herold M, et al. Utility of cardiac magnetic resonance imaging in the diagnosis of hypertrophic cardiomyopathy. Circulation 2005;112:855–61.

[33] Maron BJ, Gross BW, Stark SI. Extreme left ventricular hypertrophy. Circulation 1995;92:3748.

[34] Spirito P, Bellone P, Harris KM, et al. Magnitude of left ventricular hypertrophy predicts the risk of sudden death in hypertrophic cardiomyopathy. N Engl J Med 2000;342:1778–85.

[35] Maron BJ, Pelliccia A, Spirito P. Cardiac disease in young trained athletes: Insights into methods for distinguishing athlete's heart from structural heart disease with particular emphasis on hypertrophic cardiomyopathy. Circulation 1995;91:1596–601.

[36] Charron P, Dubourg O, Desnos M, et al. Diagnostic value of electrocardiography and echocardiography for familial hypertrophic cardiomyopathy in a genotyped adult population. Circulation 1997; 96:214–9.

[37] Roberts WC. Congenital coronary arterial anomalies unassociated with major anomalies of the heart or great vessels. In: Roberts WC, editor. Adult congenital heart disease. Philadelphia: FA Davis Co; 1987. p. 583–629.

[38] Basso C, Maron BJ, Corrado D, et al. Clinical profile of congenital coronary artery anomalies with origin from the wrong aortic sinus leading to sudden death in young competitive athletes. Circulation 1976;53:122–31.

[39] Maron BJ, Leon MB, Swain JA, et al. Prospective identification by two-dimensional echocardiography of anomalous origin of the left main coronary artery from the right sinus of valsalva. Am J Cardiol 1991; 68:140–2.

[40] Jureidini SB, Eaton C, Williams J, et al. Transthoracic two-dimensional and color flow echocardiographic diagnosis of aberrant left coronary artery. Am Heart J 1994;127:438–40.

[41] Thiene G, Nava A, Corrado D, et al. Right ventricular cardiomyopathy and sudden death in young people. N Engl J Med 1988;318:129–33.

[42] McKenna WJ, Thiene G, Nava A, et al. Diagnosis of arrhythmogenic right ventricular dysplasia/cardiomyopathy. Br Heart J 1994;71:215–8.

[43] Corrado D, Basso C, Rizzoli G, et al. Does sport activity enhance the risk of sudden death in adolescents and young adults? J Am Coll Cardiol 2003; 42:1964–6.

[44] Daliento L, Turrini P, Nava A, et al. Arrhythmogenic right ventricular cardiomyopathy in young versus adult patients: similarities and differences. J Am Coll Cardiol 1995;25:655–64.

[45] Corrado D, Basso C, Thiene G, et al. Spectrum of clinicopathologic manifestations of arrhythmogenic right ventricular cardiomyopathy/dysplasia: a multicenter study. J Am Coll Cardiol 1997;30:1512–20.

[46] Pelliccia A, Maron BJ. Preparticipation cardiovascular evaluation of the competitive athlete: Perspectives from the 30-year Italian experience. Am J Cardiol 1995;75:827–8.

[47] Corrado D, Basso C, Schiavon M, et al. Screening for hypertrophic cardiomyopathy in young athletes. N Engl J Med 1998;339:364–9.

[48] Bharti S, Lev M. Congenital abnormalities of the conduction system in sudden death in young adults. J Am Coll Cardiol 1986;8:1096–104.

[49] Schwarz ER, Klues HG, vom Dahl J, et al. Functional, angiographic and intracoronary Doppler flow characteristics in symptomatic patients with myocardial bridging: effect of short-term intravenous

beta-blocker medication. J Am Coll Cardiol 1996;27:
1637–45.

[50] Lange RA, Hillis LD. Cardiovascular complications
of cocaine use. N Engl J Med 2001;345:351–8.

[51] Samenuk D, Link MS, Homoud MK, et al. Adverse
cardiovascular events temporally associated with ma
huang, an herbal source of ephedrine. Mayo Clin
Proc 2002;77:12–6.

[52] Estes NAM III, Kloner R, Olshansky B, et al. Drugs
and performance-enhancing substances. In, 36th
Bethesda Conference. Eligibility recommendations
for competitive athletes with cardiovascular abnormalities (BJ Maron and DP Zipes). J Am Coll
Cardiol 2005;45:1368–9.

[53] Link MS, Wang PJ, Pandian NG, et al. An experimental model of sudden death due to low-energy
chest-wall impact (commotio cordis). N Engl
J Med 1998;338:1805–11.

[54] Link MS, Maron BJ, Garan AR, et al. Impact object
shape and resultant left ventricular pressure critically
important in the generation of ventricular fibrillation
from chest wall impact (commotio cordis) [abstract].
J AmColl Cardiol 2007;49(Suppl A):16A.

[55] Link MS, Maron BJ, Song CP, et al. Evidence for
mechanically-induced ion-channel dysfunction as
a mechanism in chest blow-induced ventricular
fibrillation (commotio cordis) [abstract]. J Am Coll
Cardiol 2007;49(Suppl A):7A.

[56] Link MS, Wang PJ, VanderBrink BA, et al. Selective
activation of the K^+_{ATP} channel is a mechanism by
which sudden death is produced by low energy chest
wall impact (commotio cordis). Circulation 1999;
100:413–8.

[57] Weinstock J, Maron BJ, Song C, et al. Failure of
commercially available chest wall protectors to prevent sudden cardiac death induced by chest wall
blows in an experimental model of commotio cordis.
Pediatrics 2006;117:e656–62 [1404–5].

[58] Maron BJ, Gohman TE, Aeppli D. Prevalence of
sudden cardiac death during competitive sports activities in Minnesota high school athletes. J Am
Coll Cardiol 1998;32:1881–4.

[59] Maron BJ, Poliac LC, Roberts WO. Risk for sudden
cardiac death associated with marathon running.
J Am Coll Cardiol 1996;28:428–31.

[60] Roberts WO, Maron BJ. Evidence for decreasing
occurrence of sudden cardiac death associated
with the marathon. J Am Coll Cardiol 2005;46:
1373–4.

[61] Maron BJ, Shen W-K, Link MS, et al. Efficacy of
implantable cardioverter-defibrillators for the prevention of sudden death in patients with hypertrophic cardiomyopathy. N Engl J Med 2000;342:
365–73.

[62] Maron BJ, Spirito P, Shen W-K, et al. Implantable
cardioverter-defibrillators and prevention of sudden
cardiac death in hypertropic cardiomyopathy.
JAMA 2007;298:405–12.

[63] Glover DW, Maron BJ. Profile of preparticipation
cardiovascular screening for high school athletes.
JAMA 1998;279:1817–9.

[64] Pfister GC, Puffer JC, Maron BJ. Preparticipation
cardiovascular screening for US collegiate student-
athletes. JAMA 2000;283:1597–9.

[65] Glover DW, Glover DW, Maron BJ. Evolution in
the process of screening U.S. high school student-
athletes for cardiovascualr disease. America Journal
of Cardiology, in press.

[66] Montgomery JV, Harris KM, Casey SA, et al. Relation of electrocardiographic patterns to phenotypic expression and clinical outcome in
hypertrophic cardiomyopathy. Am J Cardiol 2005;
96:270–5.

[67] Maron BJ, Spirito P, Wesley YE, et al. Development
and progression of left ventricular hypertrophy in
children with hypertrophic cardiomyopathy.
N Engl J Med 1986;315:610–4.

[68] Maron BJ, Klues HG. Surviving competitive athletics with hypertrophic cardiomyopathy. Am J Cardiol
1994;73:1098–104.

[69] Paterick TE, Paterick TJ, Fletcher GF, et al. Medical and legal issues impacting the cardiovascular
evaluation of competitive athletes. JAMA 2005;
294:3011–8.

ELSEVIER
SAUNDERS

Cardiol Clin 25 (2007) 415–422

CARDIOLOGY
CLINICS

Arrhythmogenic Right Ventricular Cardiomyopathy in Athletes: Diagnosis, Management, and Recommendations for Sport Activity

Cristina Basso, MD, PhD[a], Domenico Corrado, MD, PhD[b],
Gaetano Thiene, MD, FRCP Hon[a],*

[a]*Department of Medical-Diagnostic Sciences and Special Therapies, University of Padua Medical School,
Via A. Gabelli 61, 35121 Padova, Italy*
[b]*Department of Cardio-Thoracic and Vascular Sciences, University of Padua Medical School,
Via N. Giustiniani 2, 35128 Padova, Italy*

Arrhythmogenic right ventricular cardiomyopathy/dysplasia (ARVC/D) is an inherited heart muscle disease that predominantly affects the right ventricle and is characterized pathologically by progressive replacement of right ventricular myocardium with fibrofatty tissue [1–10]. Clinically, the disease presents with myocardial electrical instability leading to ventricular tachycardia or ventricular fibrillation which may precipitate cardiac arrest, particularly during physical exercise [11].

This article examines the role of ARVC/D in causing sudden death in young competitive athletes and suggests a prevention strategy based on identification of affected athletes at preparticipation screening. Systematic cardiovascular screening (including 12-lead ECG) of all subjects embarking in sports activity has the potential to identify those athletes at risk and to reduce mortality [12,13].

The advent of molecular genetics has provided new insights in understanding the etiopathogenesis of ARVC/D, showing that it is a desmosomal disease resulting from defective cell adhesion

proteins such as desmoplakin, plakoglobin, plakophilin-2, desmoglein-2, and desmocollin-2 [14–18]. It has been postulated that the lack of the protein or the incorporation of mutant protein into cardiac desmosomes may provoke remodeling with detachment of myocytes at the intercalated disks, particularly under the condition of mechanical stress during training and competitive sports activity [19,20]. As a consequence, there is progressive myocyte death with subsequent repair by fibrofatty replacement. Life-threatening ventricular arrhythmias such as ventricular tachycardia and fibrillation may occur during the "hot phase" of myocyte death or later in the form of a scar-related macroreentrant mechanism [21].

Arrhythmogenic right ventricular cardiomyopathy/dysplasia: a major cause of sudden death in young athletes

Systematic monitoring and pathologic investigation of sudden death in young people and athletes of the Veneto region of Italy has shown that ARVC/D is the most common pathologic substrate, accounting for nearly one fourth of fatal events on the athletic field [11,12,22]. The incidence of sudden death from ARVC/D in athletes is estimated to be 0.5 cases per 100,000 persons per year (Fig. 1). In the authors' experience, sudden death victims with ARVC/D have all been male with a mean age of 22.6 ± 4 years [22].

This work was supported by the European Commission ARVC/D Project, Brussels, Veneto Region, Venice, and Telethon, Rome; Cariparo Foundation, Pedova; Ministry of Health, Rome.

* Corresponding author.
E-mail address: gaetano.thiene@unipd.it
(G. Thiene).

cardiology.theclinics.com

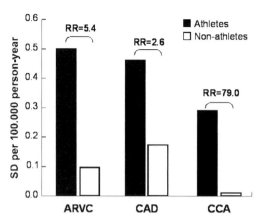

Fig. 1. Incidence and relative risk (RR) of sudden death (SD) from major cardiovascular causes among young athletes and non-athletes. CAD, coronary artery disease; CCA, congenital coronary artery anomalies. (*Modified from* Corrado D, Basso C, Rizzoli G, et al. Does sports activity enhance the risk of sudden death in adolescents and young adults? J Am Coll Cardiol 2003;42:1959–63; with permission. Copyright © 2003 American College of Cardiology Foundation.)

The hallmark lesion of the disease is extensive replacement of the right ventricular myocardium by fibrofatty tissue (Fig. 2). At autopsy, hearts demonstrate massive regional or diffuse fibrofatty infiltration, a parchment-like and translucent free wall of the right ventricle, and mild-to-moderate right ventricular dilatation, together with aneurysmal dilatations of posterobasal, apical, and outflow tract regions. These right ventricular pathologic features allow a differential diagnosis with training-induced right ventricular adaptation ("athlete's heart"), usually consisting of global right ventricular enlargement without regional dilatation or deformities. Histologically, fibrofatty infiltration is usually associated with focal myocardial necrosis and patchy inflammatory infiltrates. Fibrofatty scar and aneurysms are potential sources of life-threatening ventricular arrhythmias. The histopathologic arrangement of the surviving myocardium embedded in the replaced fibrofatty tissue may lead to inhomogeneous intraventricular conduction predisposing to reentrant mechanisms.

Although ARVC/D has been demonstrated to be the leading cause of sudden death in athletes of

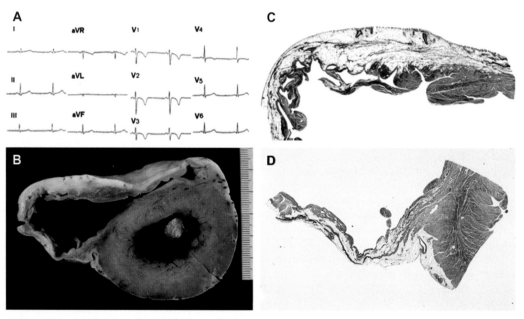

Fig. 2. Electrocardiographic and pathologic features in a 17-year-old soccer player who died suddenly of ARVC/D during a game. (*A*) Twelve-lead ECG obtained at preparticipation screening shows typical abnormalities consisting of inverted T waves from V_1 to V_4. (*B*) Transverse section of the heart specimen shows anterior and posterior aneurysms due to extreme thinning of the right ventricular free wall. (*C, D*) Panoramic histologic views of the anterior and posterior right ventricular free walls show transmural fibrofatty replacement of myocardium (Heidenhain trichrome). (*Modified from* Basso C, Thiene G, Corrado D, et al. Arrhythmogenic right ventricular cardiomyopathy. Dysplasia, dystrophy, or myocarditis? Circulation 1996;94:983–91; with permission.)

the Veneto region of Italy, studies in the United States have shown a higher prevalence of other pathologic substrates, such as hypertrophic cardiomyopathy, anomalous coronary arteries, and myocarditis [23–25].

This discrepancy may be explained by several factors. There have been no previous investigations, such as the Juvenile Sudden Death Research Project in the Veneto region of Italy, in which a consecutive series of sudden deaths in young people occurring in a well-defined geographic area have been prospectively investigated with a homogeneous ethnic group. The previously reported causes in the United States may have been influenced by the unavoidable limitations in patient selection because of retrospective analysis. Moreover, in other large studies, the autopsies were usually performed by different examiners, including local pathologists and medical coroners [25]. In the Italian study, to obtain a higher level of confidence in the results, the morphologic examination of all hearts was performed according to a standard protocol by the same group of experienced cardiovascular pathologists. Comparison between the previous and the present study with regard to the prevalence of ARVC/D among the causes of sudden death in young people and athletes is limited by the fact that ARVC/D is a clinical-pathologic condition that has been discovered only recently [2,3]. ARVC/D is rarely associated with cardiomegaly and usually spares the left ventricular function; therefore, affected hearts may be erroneously diagnosed as normal hearts [2,4,5,26]. In the past, some sudden deaths in young people and athletes in which the routine pathologic examination disclosed a normal heart may, in fact, have been due to unrecognized ARVC/D. The high incidence of ARVC/D in the Veneto region may be due to a genetic factor in the population of northeastern Italy [27]; however, ARVC/D can no longer be considered as a peculiar "Venetian disease," because there is growing evidence that it is ubiquitous, although largely underdiagnosed both clinically and at post-mortem investigation, and accounts for significant arrhythmic morbidity and mortality worldwide [28,29].

Preparticipation screening of young people embarking in competitive athletic activity, which has been practiced in Italy for more than 20 years, has changed the prevalence of pathologic substrates of sports-related sudden death. The authors recently demonstrated that sudden death from hypertrophic cardiomyopathy in athletic fields can be successfully prevented by identification and disqualification of the affected athletes at preparticipation screening [12]. As a consequence of this process, other cardiovascular conditions such as ARVC/D, congenital coronary artery anomalies, and premature coronary artery disease now account for a greater proportion of all sudden deaths in Italian athletes.

Arrhythmogenic right ventricular cardiomyopathy/dysplasia and the risk of sudden death during effort

Adolescent and young adults involved in sports activity have a 2.8 greater risk of sudden cardiovascular death than their non-athletic counterparts as demonstrated by a prospective clinicopathologic study of sudden death in the young in the Veneto region of Italy [22]. Sports, per se, is not the cause of the enhanced mortality but triggers cardiac arrest in those athletes who have morbid cardiovascular conditions (eg, cardiomyopathy, premature coronary artery disease, and congenital coronary artery anomalies) that predispose to life-threatening ventricular arrhythmias during physical exercise.

ARVC/D leads to sudden death, with an estimated 5.4 times greater risk of dying suddenly during competitive sports than during sedentary activity (Fig. 1). The reason for the propensity for ARVC/D to precipitate effort-dependent sudden cardiac arrest is not completely known. Physical exercise acutely increases right ventricular afterload and cavity enlargement which, in turn, may elicit ventricular arrhythmias by stretching the diseased right ventricular myocardium [30] or favoring reentrant arrhythmic mechanisms. Mechanical stress, such as that occurring during training and sports competition, may provoke myocyte death and associated ventricular arrhythmias in the presence of genetically defective desmosomes [19,27]. The adverse effect of exercise on the phenotypic expression of ARVC/D was recently addressed by Kirchhof and colleagues [20] in an experimental study on heterozygous plakoglobin-deficient mice. When compared with wild-type controls, mutant mice had increased right ventricular volume, reduced right ventricular function, and more frequent and severe ventricular tachycardia of right ventricular origin. Endurance training accelerated the development of right ventricular dysfunction and arrhythmias in plakoglobin-deficient mice.

Alternatively, a "denervation supersensitivity" of the right ventricle to catecholamines has been advanced to explain exercise-induced ventricular arrhythmias [31]. Sympathetic nerve trunks may be damaged or interrupted by the right ventricular fibrofatty replacement which distinctively progresses from the epicardium to the endocardium, resulting in a denervation hypersensitivity to catecholamines. Arrhythmogenic mechanisms in the denervated hypersensitive myofibers include dispersion of refractoriness and reentry, triggered activity, or both.

In a subgroup of patients with familial ARVC/D, a cardiac ryanodine receptor (RYR2) missense mutation leading to gain of function and abnormal calcium release from the sarcoplasmic reticulum has been identified [32]. Wall mechanical stress, such as that induced by right ventricular volume overload during exercise, and increased heart rate are expected to exacerbate the cardiac ryanodine channel dysfunction. A potential arrhythmogenic mechanism of sport-related cardiac arrest in patients with ARVC/D is triggered activity due to late afterdepolarizations, which are provoked by intracellular calcium overload and enhanced by adrenergic stimulation [33].

Clinical profile of athletes dying suddenly of arrhythmogenic right ventricular cardiomyopathy/dysplasia

Early identification of athletes with ARVC/D has a crucial role in the prevention of sudden death because sports' disqualification is life saving. The most frequent clinical manifestations of the disease consist of ECG depolarization/repolarization changes mainly localized to right precordial leads, global or regional morphologic and functional alterations of the right ventricle, and arrhythmias of right ventricular origin [1,2,5,9,10,34,35]. The disease should be suspected even in asymptomatic individuals on the basis of ECG abnormalities and ventricular arrhythmias [1,3,11,12]. Ultimately, the diagnosis relies on visualization of morphofunctional right ventricular abnormalities by imaging techniques (eg, echocardiography, angiography, and cardiac magnetic resonance) and, in selected cases, by histopathologic demonstration of fibrofatty substitution at endomyocardial biopsy [6–8,34]. According to the task force criteria, the diagnosis of ARVC/D is established in individuals who have two major criteria, one major and two minor criteria, or four minor criteria. Timely identification of ARVC/D is challenging in asymptomatic individuals and largely relies on familial

occurrence of the disease, the presence of ECG abnormalities, or the detection of morphologic right ventricular abnormalities with imaging techniques. The incidence of ventricular tachyarrhythmia (such as ventricular tachycardia of right ventricular origin, usually elicited by exercise) represents a substantial contribution to the clinical diagnosis of ARVC/D.

More than 80% of athletes in the Veneto region series who died of ARVC/D had a history of syncope, ECG changes, or ventricular arrhythmias (Fig. 2) [12]. More recently, the authors confirmed these findings by reviewing clinical and ECG data in a Multicenter International Registry for 22 young competitive athletes who died suddenly of ARVC/D proven at autopsy [36]. Right precordial inverted T waves (beyond lead V_1) had been recorded in 88% of the athletes who had a 12-lead ECG during life and subsequently died suddenly. The right precordial QRS duration was greater than 110 milliseconds in 76%, and ventricular arrhythmias with a left bundle branch block pattern were found in 76%, mostly in the form of isolated/coupled premature ventricular beats or nonsustained ventricular tachycardia. Limited exercise testing induced ventricular arrhythmias in 6 of 12 athletes (50%). Submaximal exercise testing, available in five athletes, showed a "pseudo" normalization of right precordial repolarization abnormalities in all. Most of the young competitive athletes who died suddenly of ARVC/D showed ECG abnormalities that could raise the suspicion of underlying cardiovascular disease at preparticipation evaluation and lead to further testing for a definitive diagnosis. Right precordial T-wave inversion (beyond V_1) appears to be the most useful clinical marker for the presence of potentially fatal ARVC/D in apparently healthy young competitive athletes, considering that T-wave inversion in V_1-V_3 occurs in less than 1% of men with apparently normal hearts who are aged 19 to 45 years [37].

Turrini and colleagues [38] retrospectively investigated the value of clinical and ECG findings in predicting the risk for sudden death in 60 patients with ARVC/D. A QRS dispersion greater than or equal to 40 milliseconds was the strongest independent predictor of sudden death with a sensitivity and specificity of 90% and 77%, respectively. Syncope, a QT dispersion less than or equal to 65 milliseconds, and negative T waves beyond V_1 refined arrhythmic risk stratification in these patients.

Preparticipation screening and prevention of sudden death

Systematic preparticipation screening based on 12-lead ECG in addition to a history and physical examination has been the practice in Italy for more than 20 years [12,13]. This screening strategy has proved to be effective in the identification of athletes with previously undiagnosed hypertrophic cardiomyopathy owing to the high sensitivity (up to 95%) of 12-lead ECG for the suspicion or detection of this condition, subsequently confirmed by two-dimensional echocardiography, in otherwise asymptomatic athletes. Moreover, during long-term follow-up, no deaths were recorded among these disqualified athletes with hypertrophic cardiomyopathy, suggesting that restriction from competition may reduce the risk of sudden death [12].

Despite the high prevalence of ECG abnormalities at preparticipation evaluation, such as T-wave inversion in right precordial leads and ventricular arrhythmias with a left bundle branch block morphology, the majority of sudden death victims from ARVC/D were not identified at preparticipation screening, explaining why this condition was previously reported to be the leading cause of sudden death in Italian athletes [12,22]. The most plausible explanation is that, unlike hypertrophic cardiomyopathy, ARVC/D is a condition that has been discovered only recently (approximately 2 decades ago); therefore, it was either underdiagnosed or regarded with skepticism by cardiologists.

Recently, the authors reported the results of a time-trend analysis of the changes in incidence rates and causes of sudden cardiovascular death in young athletes aged 12 to 35 years in the Veneto region of Italy between 1979 and 2004, after the introduction of systematic preparticipation screening [13]. Over the same time interval, a parallel study examined trends in cardiovascular causes of disqualification from competitive sports in 42,386 athletes undergoing preparticipation screening at the Center for Sports Medicine in Padua. Fifty-five sudden cardiovascular deaths occurred in screened athletes (1.9 deaths/100,000 person-years) and 265 deaths in unscreened non-athletes (0.79 deaths/100,000 person-years). The annual incidence of sudden cardiovascular death in athletes decreased by approximately 90% from 3.6 deaths per 100,000 person-years in 1979 to 1980 to 0.4 deaths per 100,000 person-years in 2001 to 2004, whereas the incidence of sudden death among the unscreened non-athletic population did not change significantly over that time. The decline in the death rate started after compulsory screening was initiated and persisted to the late screening period. When compared with the pre-screening period (1979–1981), the relative risk of sudden cardiovascular death was 44% lower in the early screening period (1982–1992) and 79% lower in the late screening period (1993–2004). Most of the reduced death rate was due to fewer cases of sudden death from cardiomyopathy, mostly from ARVC/D. Time-trend analysis showed that the incidence of sudden death from this latter condition fell by 84% over the 24-year span. This decline of mortality from cardiomyopathy paralleled the concomitant increase in the number of athletes with cardiomyopathy (both hypertrophic cardiomyopathy and ARVC/D) who were identified and disqualified from competitive sports over the screening periods at the Center for Sports Medicine in Padua. Screening athletes for cardiomyopathy is a life-saving strategy, and 12-lead ECG is a sensitive and powerful tool for the identification, risk stratification, and management of athletes affected by hypertrophic cardiomyopathy and ARVC/D [13,39].

Molecular genetics and familial investigation following the diagnosis of arrhythmogenic right ventricular cardiomyopathy/dysplasia in an athlete

Blood samples should be taken to perform a genetic analysis and a search for mutations of genes encoding for desmosomal proteins completed. In a study of 90 unrelated Italian probands, nearly half were positive for different defective proteins of a desmosomal complex [40].

Currently, no variability in risk stratification has been observed in relation to disease genes. Routine clinical evaluation of family members is mandatory and consists of physical examination, 12-lead ECG, signal-averaged ECG, 24-hour Holter ECG, and two-dimensional and Doppler echocardiography. Cardiac magnetic resonance imaging and invasive examination are performed when deemed necessary. The family members may be found to be clinically affected, clinically unaffected, or to have uncertain findings. Genetic analysis is clearly the gold standard to establish who is the carrier of the disease; however, only one third of family members with positive genetic tests fulfill the diagnostic criteria. Another 15% share some instrumental abnormalities (eg, premature ventricular beats, positive late potentials), although they are not enough to achieve the diagnosis.

The need to broaden the diagnostic criteria in relatives for familial ARVC/D has been underlined [41]. Moreover, a significant proportion of family members carry the genetic mutation but do not present with clinical signs ("healthy carriers"). This observation may be due to the young age of the subject (in whom the disease has not yet developed), the low penetrance of the gene mutation, or the low sensitivity of diagnostic tests.

If a family member who is clinically unaffected has negative results for the disease gene mutation ("noncarrier"), he or she can be considered healthy, does not need further checkups, and can be assured that they will not transmit the disease to offspring. An intriguing situation is the clinically unaffected family member carrying a disease gene mutation ("healthy carrier"). This subject must be considered potentially at risk because the disease is progressive and can appear late during life, and frequent clinical checkups are mandatory. Physical activity/competitive sports should be always forbidden considering the legal implications. Noncompetitive sports may be allowed, providing regular checkups in the follow-up.

Recommendations for sport activity in athletes affected by arrhythmogenic right ventricular cardiomyopathy/dysplasia

The ultimate diagnosis of ARVC/D in a young competitive athlete can be difficult due to the presence of physiologic (and reversible) structural and electrical adaptations of the cardiovascular system to long-term athletic training. This condition, known as athlete's heart, is characterized by an increase in ventricular cavity dimension and wall thickness that overlaps with cardiomyopathy [42]. An accurate differential diagnosis is crucial not only because of the potentially adverse outcome associated with cardiomyopathy in an athlete but also due to the possibility of misdiagnosis of pathologic conditions requiring unnecessary disqualification from sport, with financial and psychologic consequences.

A sizeable proportion of highly trained athletes have an increase in right ventricular cavity dimensions, which raises the question of ARVC/D. Morphologic criteria in favor of physiologic right ventricular enlargement consists of preserved global and regional ventricular function, without evidence of wall motion abnormalities such as dyskinetic regions or diastolic bulgings.

During the last 2 decades, advances in molecular genetics have allowed the identification of a growing number of defective genes involved in the pathogenesis of ARVC/D [27,40]. The hope is that molecular genetic tests will be available clinically in the near future for definitive differential diagnosis of ARVC/D versus training-related physiologic changes.

After ARVC/D is diagnosed in an athlete, sudden cardiac death may be prevented by different approaches (Fig. 3): (1) by avoiding the trigger, such as strenuous exercise in athletes who are identified as having the disease by clinical or genetic

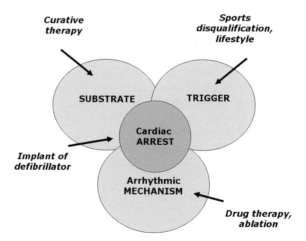

Fig. 3. Diagram showing the various levels of interventions for sudden death prevention in ARVC/D. (*Modified from* Marcus F, Nava A, Thiene G, editors. Arrhythmogenic right ventricular cardiomyopathy/dysplasia: recent advances. Milan (Italy): Springer; 2007.)

screening; (2) by preventing life-threatening arrhythmias using drug therapy or ablation; or (3) by cardioverter defibrillator implantation, an extremely effective therapy to treat life-threatening ventricular arrhythmias that can result in cardiac arrest.

All of the previously mentioned therapeutic and preventive measures are palliative and not curative. The definitive cure for the disease is still elusive. Cardiac transplantation is employed to treat end-stage cardiac failure or refractory electrical instability. Prevention of myocyte apoptotic death, inflammation, and fibrofatty replacement, the basic mechanisms of myocardial injury and repair, will require understanding the etiopathogenesis of ARVC/D.

According to US and European recommendations for sports eligibility [43,44], athletes with a clinical diagnosis of ARVC/D should be excluded from all competitive sports. This recommendation is independent of age, gender, and phenotypic appearance and does not differ for those athletes without symptoms, or for those treated with drugs, surgery, catheter ablation, or an implantable defibrillator. The presence of a free-standing automated external defibrillator at sporting events should not be considered absolute protection against sudden death [45], nor should it be considered a justification for participation in competitive sports in athletes with previously diagnosed ARVC/D [43,44,46].

References

[1] Marcus F, Nava A, Thiene G, editors. Arrhythmogenic right ventricular cardiomyopathy/dysplasia: recent advances. Milan (Italy): Springer; 2007.

[2] Marcus F, Fontaine G, Guiraudon G, et al. Right ventricular dysplasia: a report of 24 adult cases. Circulation 1982;65:384–98.

[3] Thiene G, Nava A, Corrado D, et al. Right ventricular cardiomyopathy and sudden death in young people. N Engl J Med 1988;318:129–33.

[4] Basso C, Thiene G, Corrado D, et al. Arrhythmogenic right ventricular cardiomyopathy: dysplasia, dystrophy, or myocarditis? Circulation 1996;94: 983–91.

[5] Corrado D, Basso C, Thiene G, et al. Spectrum of clinicopathologic manifestations of arrhythmogenic right ventricular cardiomyopathy/dysplasia: a multicenter study. J Am Coll Cardiol 1997;30:1512–20.

[6] Thiene G, Nava A, Angelini A, et al. Anatomoclinical aspects of arrhythmogenic right ventricular cardiomyopathy. In: Baroldi G, Camerini F, Goodwin JF, editors. Advances in cardiomyopathies. Berlin, Germany: Springer Verlag; 1990. p. 397–408.

[7] Thiene G, Basso C, Danieli GA, et al. Arrhythmogenic right ventricular cardiomyopathy: a still underrecognized clinical entity. Trends Cardiovasc Med 1997;7:84–90.

[8] Thiene G, Basso C. Arrhythmogenic right ventricular cardiomyopathy: an update. Cardiovasc Pathol 2001;10:109–17.

[9] Nava A, Bauce B, Basso C, et al. Clinical profile and long-term follow-up of 37 families with arrhythmogenic right ventricular cardiomyopathy. J Am Coll Cardiol 2000;36:2226–33.

[10] Richardson P, McKenna WJ, Bristow M, et al. Report of the 1995 WHO/ISFC Task Force on the definition and classification of cardiomyopathies. Circulation 1996;93:841–2.

[11] Corrado D, Thiene G, Nava A, et al. Sudden death in young competitive athletes: clinico-pathologic correlations in 22 cases. Am J Med 1990;89:588–96.

[12] Corrado D, Basso C, Schiavon M, et al. Screening for hypertrophic cardiomyopathy in young athletes. N Engl J Med 1998;339:364–9.

[13] Corrado D, Basso C, Pavei A, et al. Trends in sudden cardiovascular death in young competitive athletes after implementation of a preparticipation screening program. JAMA 2006;296:1593–601.

[14] McKoy G, Protonotarios N, Crosby A, et al. Identification of a deletion of plakoglobin in arrhythmogenic right ventricular cardiomyopathy with palmoplantar keratoderma and wooly hair (Naxos disease). Lancet 2000;335:2119–24.

[15] Rampazzo A, Nava A, Malacrida S, et al. Mutation in human desmoplakin domain binding to plakoglobin causes a dominant form of arrhythmogenic right ventricular cardiomyopathy. Am J Hum Genet 2002;71:1200–6.

[16] Gerull B, Heuser A, Wichter T, et al. Mutations in the desmosomal protein plakophilin-2 are common in arrhythmogenic right ventricular cardiomyopathy. Nat Genet 2004;36:1162–4.

[17] Pilichou K, Nava A, Basso C, et al. Mutations in desmoglein-2 gene are associated with arrhythmogenic right ventricular cardiomyopathy. Circulation 2006;113:1171–9.

[18] Syrris P, Ward D, Evans A, et al. Arrhythmogenic right ventricular dysplasia/cardiomyopathy associated with mutations in the desmosomal gene desmocollin-2. Am J Hum Genet 2006;79:978–84.

[19] Basso C, Czarnowska E, Barbera MD, et al. Ultrastructural evidence of intercalated disc remodelling in arrhythmogenic right ventricular cardiomyopathy: an electron microscopy investigation on endomyocardial biopsies. Eur Heart J 2006;27:1847–54.

[20] Kirchhof P, Fabritz L, Zwiener M, et al. Age- and training-dependent development of arrhythmogenic right ventricular cardiomyopathy in heterozygous plakoglobin-deficient mice. Circulation 2006;114: 1799–806.

[21] Corrado D, Leoni L, Link MS, et al. Implantable cardioverter-defibrillator therapy for prevention of sudden death in patients with arrhythmogenic right ventricular cardiomyopathy/dysplasia. Circulation 2003;108:3084–91.

[22] Corrado D, Basso C, Rizzoli G, et al. Does sports activity enhance the risk of sudden death in adolescents and young adults? J Am Coll Cardiol 2003;42:1959–63.

[23] Maron BJ, Roberts WC, McAllister MA, et al. Sudden death in young athletes. Circulation 1980; 62:218–29.

[24] Maron BJ. Sudden death in young athletes. N Engl J Med 2003;349:1064–75.

[25] Van Camp SP, Bloor CM, Mueller FO, et al. Nontraumatic sports death in high school and college athletes. Med Sci Sports Exerc 1995;27:641–7.

[26] Corrado D, Basso C, Thiene G. Sudden cardiac death in young people with apparently normal heart. Cardiovasc Res 2001;50:399–408.

[27] Corrado D, Thiene G. Arrhythmogenic right ventricular cardiomyopathy/dysplasia: clinical impact of molecular genetic studies. Circulation 2006;113:1634–7.

[28] Basso C, Wichter T, Danieli GA, et al. Arrhythmogenic right ventricular cardiomyopathy: clinical registry, tissue and DNA bank. Eur Heart J 2004;25:531–4.

[29] Marcus F, Towbin JA, Zareba W, et al. ARVD/C Investigators. Arrhythmogenic right ventricular dysplasia/cardiomyopathy (ARVD/C): a multidisciplinary study. Design and protocol. Circulation 2003; 107:2975–8.

[30] Douglas PS, O'Toole ML, Hiller WDB, et al. Different effects of prolonged exercise on the right and left ventricles. J Am Coll Cardiol 1990;15:64–9.

[31] Wichter T, Hindricks G, Lerch H, et al. Regional myocardial sympathetic dysinnervation in arrhythmogenic right ventricular cardiomyopathy. Circulation 1994;89:667–83.

[32] Tiso N, Stephan DA, Nava A, et al. Identification of mutations in the cardiac ryanodine receptor gene in families affected with arrhythmogenic right ventricular cardiomyopathy type 2 (ARVD2). Hum Mol Genet 2001;10:189–94.

[33] Priori SG, Napolitano C, Tiso N, et al. Mutations in the cardiac ryanodine receptor gene (Rryr2) underlie catecholaminergic polymorphic ventricular tachycardia. Circulation 2000;103:196–200.

[34] McKenna WJ, Thiene G, Nava A, et al. Diagnosis of arrhythmogenic right ventricular dysplasia/cardiomyopathy. Task Force of the Working Group Myocardial and Pericardial Disease of the European Society of Cardiology and of the Scientific Council on Cardiomyopathies of the International Society and Federation of Cardiology. Br Heart J 1994;71: 215–8.

[35] Corrado D, Basso C, Thiene G. Arrhythmogenic right ventricular cardiomyopathy: diagnosis, prognosis, and treatment. Heart 2000;83:588–95.

[36] Corrado D, Basso C, Fontaine G, et al. Clinical profile of young competitive athletes who died suddenly

[37] Marcus FI. Prevalence of T-wave inversion beyond V1 in young normal individuals and usefulness for the diagnosis of arrhythmogenic right ventricular cardiomyopathy/dysplasia. Am J Cardiol 2005;95: 1070–1.

[38] Turrini P, Corrado D, Basso C, et al. Dispersion of ventricular depolarization-repolarization: a noninvasive marker for risk stratification in arrhythmogenic right ventricular cardiomyopathy. Circulation 2001;103:3075–80.

[39] Corrado D, Pelliccia A, Bjornstad HH, et al. Cardiovascular pre-participation screening of young competitive athletes for prevention of sudden death: proposal for a common European protocol. Consensus Statement of the Study Group of Sport Cardiology of the Working Group of Cardiac Rehabilitation and Exercise Physiology and the Working Group of Myocardial and Pericardial Diseases of the European Society of Cardiology. Eur Heart J 2005;26:516–24.

[40] Rampazzo A, Danieli GA. Advances in genetics: dominant forms. In: Marcus FI, Nava A, Thiene G, editors. Arrhythmogenic right ventricular cardiomyopathy/dysplasia – Recent advances. Springer, Milano; 2007. p. 7–14.

[41] Hamid MS, Norman M, Quraishi A, et al. Prospective evaluation of relatives for familial arrhythmogenic right ventricular cardiomyopathy/dysplasia reveals a need to broaden diagnostic criteria. J Am Coll Cardiol 2002;40:1445–50.

[42] Maron BJ, Pelliccia A, Spirito P. Cardiac disease in young trained athletes: insights into methods for distinguishing athlete's heart from structural heart disease, with particular emphasis on hypertrophic cardiomyopathy. Circulation 1995;91:1596–601.

[43] Maron BJ, Zipes DP. 36th Bethesda Conference: recommendations for determining eligibility for competition in athletes with cardiovascular abnormalities. J Am Coll Cardiol 2005;45:1373–5.

[44] Pelliccia A, Fagard R, Bjornstad HH, et al. Recommendations for competitive sports participation in athletes with cardiovascular disease: a consensus document from the Study Group of Sports Cardiology of the Working Group of Cardiac Rehabilitation and Exercise Physiology and the Working Group of Myocardial and Pericardial Diseases of the European Society of Cardiology. Eur Heart J 2005;26:1422–45.

[45] Drezner JA, Rogers KJ. Sudden cardiac arrest in intercollegiate athletes: detailed analysis and outcomes of resuscitation in nine cases. Heart Rhythm 2006;3:755–9.

[46] Maron BJ, Chaitman BR, Ackerman MJ, et al. Recommendations for physical activity and recreational sports participation for young patients with genetic cardiovascular diseases. Circulation 2004;109: 2807–16.

Myocarditis and Dilated Cardiomyopathy in Athletes: Diagnosis, Management, and Recommendations for Sport Activity

Cristina Basso, MD, PhD[a],*, Elisa Carturan, BSc, PhD[a],
Domenico Corrado, MD, PhD[b],
Gaetano Thiene, MD, FRCP Hon[a]

[a]Department of Medical-Diagnostic Sciences and Special Therapies, University of Padua Medical School,
Via A. Gabelli 61, 35121 Padova, Italy
[b]Department of Cardio-Thoracic and Vascular Sciences, University of Padua Medical School, Via N. Giustiniani 2,
35128 Padova, Italy

According to the World Health Organization/ International Society and Federation of Cardiology Task Force on the Definition and Classification of Cardiomyopathies, "myocarditis is an inflammatory heart muscle disease associated with cardiac dysfunction and it is diagnosed by established histological, immunological, and immunohistochemical criteria." It is characterized by the histologic evidence of inflammatory infiltrates associated with myocyte degeneration and necrosis of nonischemic origin [1]. Currently, it is listed among specific cardiomyopathies and, as such, called inflammatory cardiomyopathy [2].

Myocarditis may be classified based on etiologic (infective or noninfective myocarditis) and histologic criteria (lymphocytic, eosinophilic, polymorphous, granulomatous, giant cell). Among noninfective forms of myocarditis, the hypersensitivity type is the most common form of acute drug-related myocardial injury. The histopathology is characterized by a diffuse inflammatory infiltrate rich in eosinophils. In contrast, toxic myocarditis consists of myocyte necrosis associated with a mixed inflammatory infiltrate of polymorphonuclear and mononuclear cells.

Several medications and toxins may exert a direct cytotoxic effect on the heart (eg, lithium, doxorubicin, cocaine, catecholamines, acetaminophen), as well as environmental toxins (lead, arsenic, alcohol, carbon monoxide) or wasp, scorpion, and spider stings; however, infectious agents, such as viruses, are the most common cause of myocarditis. Infectious causes most commonly include viral (coxsackievirus, adenovirus, parvovirus, herpes virus, HIV), bacterial (diphtheria, meningococcus, psittacosis, streptococcus), rickettsial (typhus, Rocky Mountain spotted fever), fungal (aspergillosis, candidiasis), and parasitic agents (Chagas disease, toxoplasmosis) [3]. Acute myocarditis, especially viral forms, can be resolved without sequela; however, progression in the chronic form (ie, dilated cardio myopathy [DCM]) is not a rare event.

The diagnosis of myocarditis relies on established histopathologic, histochemical, or molecular criteria but is clinically challenging. The clinical presentation of myocarditis is highly variable and includes unexplained congestive heart failure (eg, exertional dyspnea, fatigue) or cardiogenic shock, chest pain with myocardial enzyme release mimicking myocardial infarction, palpitations, syncope, or even sudden death. The clinical evaluation of patients with suspected myocarditis includes a personal and family history, physical examination, 12-lead ECG, and echocardiography. Additional testing (such as 24-hour ECG

This work was supported by the Veneto Region, Venice, Italy; Cariparo Foundation, Pedove, Italy; Ministry of Health, Rome, Italy.

* Corresponding author.
E-mail address: cristina.basso@unipd.it (C. Basso).

monitoring) may be required according to the specific case.

Evidence of fever and flulike illness, or circumstances supporting previous viral infection should be investigated. The ECG changes include frequent, complex ventricular, or supraventricular arrhythmias, ST-T segment alteration (usually depression), T-wave inversion, and conduction abnormalities, mainly left bundle branch or atrioventricular blocks [4].

Global left ventricular enlargement and dysfunction are usually evident by echocardiography [5]; however, localized wall motion abnormalities, mild enlargement of the left ventricular cavity, and borderline depression of systolic function are common. Tissue Doppler imaging may be useful to detect regional abnormalities of left ventricular relaxation suggestive of the presence of inflammatory lesions [6]. Modest pericardial effusion and increased reflectivity of the pericardial leaflets may be observed.

When myocarditis is suspected from the clinical profile, an endomyocardial biopsy represents the gold standard for the diagnosis by showing the inflammatory infiltrate and necrosis (ie, the Dallas criteria) [1]; however, its diagnostic accuracy is limited by low sensitivity and the high prevalence of false-negative histologic results. To increase the diagnostic sensitivity of histology, use of immunohistochemistry including a large panel of monoclonal and polyclonal antibodies is mandatory to identify and characterize the inflammatory infiltrate: CD45 (common leukocyte antigen), CD43 (T lymphocytes), CD45RO (activated T lymphocytes), CD68 (macrophages), CD20 (B lymphocytes), CD4 (T helper), and CD8 (cytotoxic T lymphocytes). The diagnostic yield of endomyocardial biopsy can be further enhanced by routine molecular analysis with DNA-RNA extraction and polymerase chain reaction (PCR) and reverse transcriptase amplification of the viral genome [7,8].

Dilated cardiomyopathy

DCM is a heart muscle disease characterized by left ventricular dilatation and systolic dysfunction with normal left ventricular wall thickness [9]. The estimated prevalence of DCM is 1 case per 2500 population, and it is the third most common cause of heart failure and one of the major diseases requiring cardiac transplantation. DCM is a heterogeneous disease with a multifactorial pathogenesis [2,10]. It may be familial/genetic, viral, or immune related, which explains why it has been listed among *primary cardiomyopathies, mixed* type in the recent statement of the American Heart Association on contemporary definitions and classification of the cardiomyopathies [2,10–12]. Autoimmunity is recognized to have a pivotal role in the pathogenesis of a substantial proportion of cases, possibly triggered by various causes of cardiac injury in genetically predisposed individuals [9,11].

The DCM phenotype with sporadic occurrence derives from a broad range of causes including infectious agents, particularly viruses, often producing myocarditis, and bacterial, fungal rickettsial, myobacterial, and parasitic agents. Two different theories have been proposed to explain myocyte damage and the progression from acute myocarditis to DCM—autoimmunity and direct cytotoxicity due to persistent viral infection. Other causes include toxins, chronic excessive consumption of alcohol, chemotherapeutic agents (anthracyclines), metals and other compounds (cobalt, lead, mercury, and arsenic), autoimmune and systemic disorders (including collagen vascular disorders), pheochromocytoma, neuromuscular disorders such as Duchenne/Becker and Emery-Dreifuss muscular dystrophies, and mitochondrial, metabolic, endocrine, and nutritional disorders (carnitine, selenium deficiencies) [12].

Approximately 20% to 35% of DCM cases have been reported as familial, with incomplete and age-dependent penetrance. The predominant mode of inheritance for DCM is autosomal dominant, with X-linked autosomal recessive and mitochondrial inheritance less frequent. Several of the mutant genes linked to autosomal dominant DCM encode contractile sarcomeric proteins (α-cardiac actin; α-tropomyosin; cardiac troponin T, I, and C; β- and α-myosin heavy chain; myosin binding protein C). Z-disc protein-encoding genes, including those for muscle LIM protein, α-actinin-2, ZASP, and titin, also have been identified. Moreover, DCM can be caused by several mutations in genes encoding cytoskeletal/sarcolemmal, nuclear envelope, sarcomere, and transcriptional coactivator proteins. The most common of these is the lamin A/C gene, also associated with conduction system disease, which encodes a nuclear envelope intermediate filament protein. Mutations in this gene also cause Emery-Dreifuss muscular dystrophy. The X-linked gene responsible for Emery-Dreifuss muscular dystrophy, which encodes for emerin (another nuclear lamin protein), also causes similar clinical features. Other DCM genes include desmin, caveolin, and α- and β-sarcoglycan, as well as the mitochondrial respiratory chain genes. X-linked DCM is caused by the Duchenne muscular dystrophy (dystrophin) gene, whereas G 4.5 (tafazzin), a mitochondrial protein of unknown function, causes Barth syndrome, which is an X-linked cardioskeletal myopathy in infants [12].

From a pathology viewpoint, hearts with DCM present grossly with left or biventricular eccentric hypertrophy due to an increase in myocardial mass and a reduction in ventricular wall thickness (in the absence of coronary, valvular, and systemic disease). At histologic examination, there is evidence of myocyte hypertrophy, attenuated myocytes with perinuclear halo due to myofibril loss, and hyperchromatic bizarrely shaped nuclei. Some inflammatory cells, mostly T lymphocytes and macrophages, are often visible, and spots of replacement-type fibrosis are present in about one third of cases.

From a clinical viewpoint, DCM may manifest at any age, most commonly in the third or fourth decade but also in young children, and usually is identified when associated with severe limiting symptoms and disability. DCM leads to progressive heart failure due to impairment of left ventricular systolic function, arrhythmias, conduction system disturbances, thromboembolism, and sudden or heart failure–related death. Although uncommon, DCM may represent a cause of arrhythmic sudden death in young/adult individuals engaged in sport activities. In family screening studies with echocardiography, asymptomatic or mildly symptomatic relatives may be identified.

The clinical evaluation of athletes with suspected DCM includes a personal and family history, physical examination, 12-lead ECG, echocardiography, and Holter monitoring. Twelve-lead ECG and Holter monitoring may reveal supraventricular and ventricular tachyarrhythmias in a very early stage of the disease, as well major conduction delays (ie, left bundle branch block and atrioventricular block).

At echocardiography, a disproportionate enlargement of the left ventricular cavity with respect to normal or mildly increased left ventricular wall thickness is typical. The left ventricular shape becomes spherical, and the mitral annulus may enlarge, resulting in valve regurgitation [13]. The ejection fraction is diminished ($<50\%$), segmental wall motion abnormalities may be present, stroke volume is reduced, and end-diastolic chamber pressure is increased. Cardiopulmonary testing may be useful to assess the impairment in physical

capacity and the occurrence of exercise-induced supraventricular/ventricular arrhythmias [14].

According to Pelliccia and colleagues [15], the differential diagnosis with physiologic left ventricular enlargement in trained athletes, mostly engaged in aerobic disciplines (eg, cycling, cross-country skiing, rowing, long-distance running), is based on the presence of normal left ventricular systolic function, no segmental wall motion abnormalities, and normal left ventricular diastolic filling (by Doppler imaging) and tissue doppler imaging pattern. Indeed, left ventricular cavity dilation in normal athletes is associated with superior physical performance as assessed by cardiopulmonary testing.

In selected athletes, left ventricular chamber dilation is associated with only a mildly reduced ejection fraction (ie, $50\%–60\%$). In these cases, it may be useful to assess the patient by echocardiography or radionuclide imaging regardless of whether a significant raise of the ejection fraction ($>60\%$) is induced during exercise. The absence of significant improvement at peak exercise suggests pathologic left ventricular dilatation.

Myocarditis and dilated cardiomyopathy as causes of sudden death in young athletes

Myocarditis has been traditionally considered an important cause of sudden death in young individuals including athletes, although its importance may be exaggerated because of overinterpretation of histologic data and the lack of standardized morphologic criteria (Fig. 1). It has been shown that intense physical exercise, either as a single episode of exhausting exercise or as persistent overtraining, can increase the susceptibility to upper respiratory infections as a consequence of a depressant effect upon T lymphocytes, interleukin, and the natural killer cell system [16]. Moreover, experimental evidence suggests that exercise during the early phase of myocarditis may increase the viral replication rate within myocytes, resulting in increased cytolysis and an enhanced immune response leading to increased inflammation and necrosis [17–19].

Sudden death may occur in the active or healed phases of myocarditis as a consequence of life-threatening ventricular arrhythmias, which develop mostly in the setting of an unstable myocardial substrate, namely inflammatory infiltrate, interstitial edema, myocardial necrosis, and fibrosis. The gross appearance of the heart is not distinctive, and its weight may be within

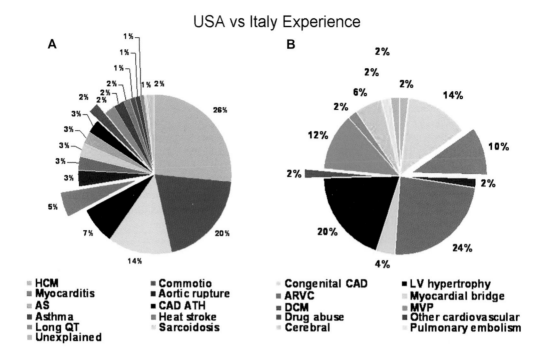

Fig. 1. Cardiovascular causes of sudden death in competitive athletes, United States (*A*) and Italy (*B*). Note the prevalence of myocarditis and DCM. ARVC, arrhythmogenic right ventricular cardiomyopathy; AS, aortic stenosis; CAD ATH, otherosclerotic coronary artery disease; HCM, hypertrophic cardiomyopathy; LV, left ventricular; MVP, mitral valve prolapse. (*Data from Refs.* [21,22].)

normal values (the "grossly normal heart" in Fig. 2) [20,21]. A patchy inflammatory infiltrate in the form of a starry sky–like feature (<14 leucocytes/mm²) and not necessarily associated with myocyte necrosis is a frequent observation. This subtle substrate, together with the possible inflammatory involvement of the conduction system, seems highly arrhythmogenic and may account for unexpected arrhythmic cardiac arrest [20].

A review of major autopsy series of sudden death in the young demonstrated that myocarditis accounted for up to 42% of fatal events [20]. This high incidence represents the strongest evidence that subclinical myocarditis can be a cause of ventricular fibrillation and come from an autopsy series on US Air Force recruits [22].

In the United States, the high-visibility tragedies of Hank Gathers and Reggie Lewis concerning competitive athletes who died suddenly were consistent with myocarditis [23]. In a recent large US series of 387 competitive young athletes who died suddenly, 20 (5.2%) showed a typical presentation of myocarditis [24].

A recent population-based study of trends in sudden cardiovascular death in an athletic and non-athletic population aged 12 to 35 years in the Veneto region of Italy demonstrated that myocarditis accounted for 13% and 15% of fatal events, respectively [25]. This rate signifies an incidence of 0.24 cases per 100,000 athlete-years. Although myocarditis in athletes is usually triggered by a viral infection, other causes such as long-term cocaine abuse can result in a similar clinical and pathologic profile [26].

Chlamydia pneumoniae was implicated as the cause of myocarditis and sudden death in 16 young Swedish elite orienteers (mean age, 25 years; 15 males/1 female) who died unexpectedly [27]. Subsequently, the investigation was extended to five other Swedish orienteers, identifying *C pneumoniae* in one, *Bartonella quintana* in two, and *Bartonella henselae* in the remaining three cases [28]. *Rickettsia helvetica* was associated with sudden death in two young Swedish men who died during exercise and who showed signs of perimyocarditis at histology [29].

In contrast, DCM is an extremely rare cause of sudden death in the athlete, being responsible for only a small minority of cardiac arrests in published series. In the Minneapolis Heart

Foundation Registry, DCM accounted for 2.3% of sudden deaths in young athletes [24]. Similarly, only 1 of 55 competitive athletes dying suddenly in the Veneto region had pathologic evidence of DCM (2%) (see Fig. 1) [30].

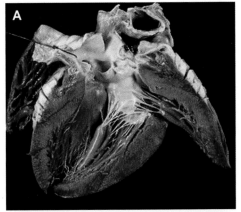

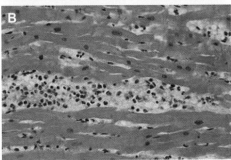

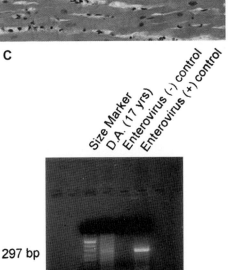

297 bp

Recommendations for sport activity in athletes affected by myocarditis and dilated cardiomyopathy

The recommendations for sport activity discussed herein are based on recent consensus documents of expert panels of the European Society of Cardiology and the Sports Cardiology Section of the European Association of Cardiovascular Prevention and Rehabilitation [31,32].

Myocarditis may evolve into a chronic inflammation, often with a subclinical course, and eventually progress into DCM (Fig. 3). It is of utmost importance to respect an adequate period of athletic rest until the disease has completely resolved. Athletes with a clinical diagnosis of myocarditis should be temporarily excluded from competitive and amateur-leisure time sport activity. This recommendation is independent of age and gender and does not differ for athletes with only mild symptoms or under treatment with drugs. After resolution of the clinical presentation (at least 6 months after the onset of the disease), clinical reassessment is indicated before the athlete re-enters a competitive sport lifestyle. Moreover, preparticipation screening should be performed every 6 months during the follow-up.

Athletes with a clinical diagnosis of DCM should be excluded from most competitive sports, with the possible exception of those of low intensity. This recommendation is independent of age, gender, and phenotypic appearance, and does not differ for those athletes without symptoms, those with prior treatment with drugs or major interventions with surgery, or those with an implantable defibrillator. Moreover, the presence of a free-standing automated external defibrillator at sporting events should not be considered absolute protection against sudden death or

Fig. 2. Sudden cardiac death in a previously asymptomatic 17-year-old boy due to acute myocarditis. (*A*) The heart specimen removed at autopsy appears grossly normal. (*B*) Histologic examination shows a polymorphous inflammatory infiltrate associated with myocyte necrosis (hematoxylin–eosin). (*C*) Agarose gel electrophoresis showing enteroviral RT-PCR results: lane 1, DNA molecular weight marker; lane 2, RT-PCR amplified products of patient's specimen; lane 3, negative control; lane 4, RT-PCR amplified products of positive control. (*Adapted from* Basso C, Calabrese F, Corrado D, et al. Postmortem diagnosis in sudden cardiac death victims: macroscopic, microscopic and molecular findings. Cardiovasc Res 2001;50:293; with permission.)

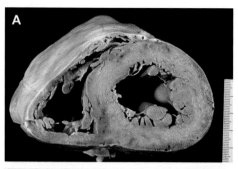

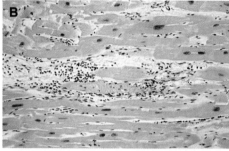

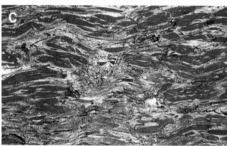

Fig. 3. Sudden cardiac death in a previously asymptomatic 21-year-old male competitive athlete due to chronic myocarditis. (A) Cross section of the heart removed at autopsy shows eccentric hypertrophy with ventricular chamber dilatation. (B) Histologic examination shows lymphocytic infiltrate associated with myocyte necrosis (hematoxylin–eosin). (C) Areas of replacement-type fibrosis are also visible (Heidenhain trichrome).

a treatment strategy for DCM, nor should it be considered a justification for participation in competitive sports in athletes with previously diagnosed DCM.

References

[1] Aretz HT, Billingham ME, Edwards WD, et al. Myocarditis: a histopathologic definition and classification. Am J Cardiovasc Pathol 1987;1:3–14.

[2] Richardson P, McKenna W, Bristow M, et al. Report of the 1995 World Health Organization/International Society and Federation of Cardiology Task Force on the Definition and Classification of Cardiomyopathies. Circulation 1996;93:841–2.

[3] Calabrese F, Thiene G. Myocarditis and inflammatory cardiomyopathy: microbiological and molecular biological aspects. Cardiovasc Res 2003;60: 11–25.

[4] Morgera T, Di Lenarda A, Dreas L, et al. Electrocardiography of myocarditis revisited: clinical and prognostic significance of electrocardiographic changes. Am Heart J 1992;124:455–66.

[5] Pianamonti B, Albed E, Cigalotto A, et al. Echocardiographic findings in myocarditis. Am J Cardiol 1988;62:2285–91.

[6] Urhausen A, Kindermann M, Bohm M, et al. Images in cardiovascular medicine: diagnosis of myocarditis by cardiac tissue velocity imaging in an Olympic athlete. Circulation 2003;108:e21–2.

[7] Martin AB, Webber S, Fricker FJ, et al. Acute myocarditis rapid diagnosis by PCR in children. Circulation 1994;90:330–9.

[8] Caforio AL, Calabrese F, Angelini A, et al. A prospective study of biopsy-proven myocarditis: prognostic relevance of clinical and aetiopathogenetic features at diagnosis. Eur Heart J 2007;28: 1326–33.

[9] Burkett E, Hershberger RE. State of the art: clinical and genetic issues in familial dilated cardiomyopathy. J Am Coll Cardiol 2005;45:969–81.

[10] Mestroni L, Rocco C, Gregori D, et al. Familial dilated cardiomyopathy: evidence for genetic and phenotypic heterogeneity. Heart Muscle Disease Study Group. J Am Coll Cardiol 1999;34:181–90.

[11] Caforio AL, Keeling PJ, Zachara E, et al. Evidence from family studies for autoimmunity in dilated cardiomyopathy. Lancet 1994;344:773–7.

[12] Maron BJ, Towbin JA, Thiene G, et al. American Heart Association; Council on Clinical Cardiology, Heart Failure and Transplantation Committee; Quality of Care and Outcomes Research and Functional Genomics and Translational Biology Interdisciplinary Working Groups; Council on Epidemiology and Prevention. Contemporary definitions and classification of the cardiomyopathies: an American Heart Association Scientific Statement from the Council on Clinical Cardiology, Heart Failure and Transplantation Committee; Quality of Care and Outcomes Research and Functional Genomics and Translational Biology Interdisciplinary Working Groups; and Council on Epidemiology and Prevention. Circulation 2006;113:1807–16.

[13] Gavazzi A, De Maria R, Renosto G, et al. The spectrum of left ventricular size in dilated cardiomyopathy: clinical correlates and prognostic implications. Am Heart J 1993;125:410–22.

[14] Mahon NG, Sharma S, Elliott PM, et al. Abnormal cardiopulmonary exercise variables in asymptomatic relatives of patients with dilated cardiomyopathy who have left ventricular enlargement. Heart 2000;83:511–7.

[15] Pelliccia A, Culasso F, Di Paolo FM, et al. Physiologic left ventricular cavity dilatation in elite athletes. Ann Intern Med 1999;130:23–31.

[16] Shephard RJ, Shek PN. Infectious diseases in athletes: new interest for an old problem. J Sports Med Phys Fitness 1994;34:11–22.

[17] Gatmaitan BG, Chason JL, Lerner AM. Augmentation of the virulence of murine coxsackievirus B3 myocardiopathy by exercise. J Exp Med 1970;131:1121–36.

[18] Ilback NG, Fohlman J, Friman G. Exercise in coxsackie B3 myocarditis: effects on heart lymphocyte subpopulations and the inflammatory reaction. Am Heart J 1989;117:1298–302.

[19] Friman G, Wesslen L. Special feature for the Olympics. Effects of exercise on the immune system: infections and exercise in high performance athletes. Immunol Cell Biol 2000;78:510–22.

[20] Basso C, Calabrese F, Corrado D, et al. Postmortem diagnosis in sudden cardiac death victims: macroscopic, microscopic and molecular findings. Cardiovasc Res 2001;50:290–300.

[21] Corrado D, Basso C, Thiene G. Sudden cardiac death in young people with apparently normal heart. Cardiovasc Res 2001;50:399–408.

[22] Phillips M, Robinowitz M, Higgins JR, et al. Sudden cardiac death in Air Force recruits: a 20-year review. JAMA 1986;256:2696–9.

[23] Maron BJ. Sudden death in young athletes: lessons from the Hank Gathers affair. N Engl J Med 1993;329:55–7.

[24] Maron BJ. Sudden death in young athletes. N Engl J Med 2003;349:1064–75.

[25] Corrado D, Basso C, Pavei A, et al. Trends in sudden cardiovascular death in young competitive athletes after implementation of a preparticipation screening program. JAMA 2006;296:1593–601.

[26] Chimenti C, Pieroni M, Frustaci A. Myocarditis: when to suspect and how to diagnose it in athletes. J Cardiovasc Med 2006;7:301–6.

[27] Wesslen L, Pahlson C, Friman G, et al. Myocarditis caused by *Chlamydia pneumoniae* (TWAR) and sudden unexpected death in a Swedish elite orienteer. Lancet 1992;340:427–8.

[28] Wesslen L, Ehrenborg C, Holmberg M, et al. Subacute bartonella infection in Swedish orienteers succumbing to sudden unexpected cardiac death or having malignant arrhythmias. Scand J Infect Dis 2001;33:429–38.

[29] Nilsson K, Lindquist O, Pahlson C. Association of *Rickettsia helvetica* with chronic perimyocarditis in sudden cardiac death. Lancet 1999;354:1169–73.

[30] Corrado D, Basso C, Rizzoli G, et al. Does sports activity enhance the risk of sudden death in adolescents and young adults? J Am Coll Cardiol 2003;42:1964–6.

[31] Pelliccia A, Fagard R, Bjornstad HH, et al. Recommendations for competitive sports participation in athletes with cardiovascular disease: a consensus document from the Study Group of Sports Cardiology of the Working Group of Cardiac Rehabilitation and Exercise Physiology and the Working Group of Myocardial and Pericardial Diseases of the European Society of Cardiology. Eur Heart J 2005;26:1422–45.

[32] Pelliccia A, Corrado D, Bjornstad HH, et al. Recommendations for participation in competitive sport and leisure-time physical activity in individuals with cardiomyopathies, myocarditis and pericarditis. Eur J Cardiovasc Prev Rehabil 2006;13:876–85.

CARDIOLOGY
CLINICS

Cardiol Clin 25 (2007) 431–440

The Athlete's Heart 2007: Diseases of the Coronary Circulation

Aaron L. Baggish, MD[a], Paul D. Thompson, MD[b],*

[a]Department of Cardiology, Massachusetts General Hospital, 55 Fruit Street, Boston, MA 02114, USA
[b]Department of Cardiology, Henry Low Heart Center, Hartford Hospital, 7th floor Jefferson, 80 Seymour Street, Hartford, CT 06102, USA

Vigorous physical exercise increases skeletal muscle oxygen requirements, which are satisfied primarily by an increase in cardiac output. This increase in cardiac output requires an augmentation in myocardial function that is in turn dependent upon a healthy coronary arterial circulation. Abnormalities in the coronary artery circulation may limit myocardial blood flow, producing exertional myocardial ischemia and diminished peak cardiac output. Coronary artery pathology can also produce acute coronary events, such as myocardial infarction and sudden death. This article discusses diseases of the coronary circulation relevant to athletes.

Normal coronary arterial circulation: embryology, anatomy, function

During embryogenesis, the two main truck coronary arteries arise as small buds (termed anlagen) from the aortic root. These buds enlarge and advance over the epicardial surface as the heart continues to develop into the adult shape. These premature arteries soon begin branching into secondary vessels, and then ultimately fuse with a pre-existing capillary network that enshrouds the fetal heart [1]. The mature coronary arterial circulation is ultimately formed through a process of capillary apoptosis and selective aggregation [2]. Though mechanisms remain incompletely understood, deviations from the normal embryonic process of coronary artery development result in the congenital coronary pathologies discussed below.

The normal coronary circulation is comprised of three distinct arteries, each responsible for blood supply to a specific portion of the ventricular myocardium. The left and right main coronary arteries originate from their respective sinuses of Valsalva behind the adjacent leaflets of the aortic valve. The right coronary artery extends over the right atrioventricular groove (right ventricular and inferior left ventricular blood supply), terminating in the posterior descending artery (posterior left ventricular blood supply) in the majority of individuals. The left main coronary artery bifurcates 2 mm to 10 mm beyond its aortic root origin into the left circumflex artery (lateral left ventricular blood supply) and the left anterior descending artery (anterior left ventricular blood supply).

The primary function of the coronary arteries is to provide oxygen and energy-rich blood to the myocardium. Myocardial perfusion, and thus substrate delivery, occurs largely during cardiac diastole. Unlike skeletal muscle, the myocardium extracts the majority of oxygen delivered even at basal levels of function. Consequently, an increase in myocardial function cannot be accommodated by increased substrate extraction and is dependent upon increased blood flow. This is accomplished by the remarkable vasodilatory capacity of the coronary circulation, which can increase blood supply four to five times the basal rate to meet increased myocardial oxygen demand [3]. Numerous complementary mechanisms, including autonomic nervous system input and the production

* Corresponding author.
E-mail address: pthomps@harthosp.org
(P.D. Thompson).

of local vasoactive metabolites, facilitate this vasodilatory response [4,5].

Coronary artery pathology: general overview

For the purpose of this review, the authors have divided coronary artery pathology (CAP) into congenital or primary CAP, and acquired or secondary CAP (Box 1). Primary CAP includes anomalies of coronary artery origin and course, whereas secondary CAP encompasses a variety of antenatal processes that compromise coronary function. Primary CAP is most frequently encountered in children and adolescents, whereas secondary CAP often presents in older individuals. This age predilection is useful in the initial assessment of a patient with suspected CAP, but clinicians must be aware that deviations from this rule are not uncommon.

Clinically relevant CAP shares the common pathophysiologic endpoint of myocardial ischemia. Myocardial ischemia is a function of both supply and demand. Athletes are particularly susceptible to even minimal coronary artery abnormalities because they frequently perform activities that markedly increase myocardial oxygen demand. Coronary artery dilation and increased myocardial perfusion normally occur in proportion to myocardial oxygen demand. Any fixed or dynamic compromise in coronary blood flow can produce myocardial ischemia that may present with such symptoms as typical chest discomfort, diaphoresis, nausea, arrhythmia, and the consequences of myocardial pump inadequacy, such as transient exercise intolerance, syncope, or heart failure.

Primary coronary artery pathology: congenital anomalies of the coronary circulation

Congenital anomalies of the coronary artery circulation account for approximately 15% to 20% of sudden death among athletes [6–8]. These abnormalities can be divided into disorders of coronary artery origin and disorders of coronary course. Sudden death caused by a coronary artery anomaly is most commonly attributed to transient myocardial ischemia occurring during vigorous physical exertion. Not all coronary circulation anomalies have the propensity to cause myocardial ischemia. The following discussion will focus on those anomalous conditions that have been associated with exertional myocardial ischemia and resultant sudden death in athletic individuals.

Anomalous coronary artery origin

In the vast majority of individuals, the proximal coronary circulation consists of a left main coronary artery and a right coronary artery that both begin within their respective sinuses of Valsalva. Any deviation from this normal anatomy is considered anomalous coronary artery origin. A comprehensive classification scheme addressing the anatomic variations of coronary arterial origin has been described by Roberts [9].

The true prevalence of anomalous coronary artery origin and the quantitative risk of sudden death associated with specific anomalous circulatory patterns are unknown. In a population of symptomatic adults referred for coronary angiography, coronary circulation anomalies were detected in approximately 0.5% of individuals [10]. The investigators provided no data on the clinical outcomes of these patients. In this report, the most common anomalous coronary abnormality was separate ostia for the left anterior descending and left circumflex arteries from the left sinus of Valsalva. In the majority of these cases, this anomaly lacks functional significance because each artery originates from an adequately developed ostium and follows a relatively normal trajectory.

There are sparse data on the prevalence of anomalous coronary artery origin in athletes.

Box 1. Important causes of coronary artery pathology in athletes

A. Primary coronary artery pathology:
   1. Anomalous coronary artery origin
      a. Left main coronary right sinus origin
      b. Left main coronary pulmonary artery origin
   2. Myocardial bridging
B. Secondary coronary artery pathology:
   1. Atherosclerotic coronary artery disease
   2. Spontaneous coronary artery dissection
      a. Peripartum period associated
      b. Connective tissue disorders
      c. Idiopathic
   3. Coronary artery vasospasm
      a. In the absence of atherosclerotic coronary disease
      b. In association with atherosclerotic coronary disease

Pelliccia and colleagues [11] used two-dimensional echocardiography in 1360 national caliber Italian athletes to screen for anomalies of coronary artery origin. Among the 1273 individuals with technically satisfactory images, 6 out of 1273 (0.5%) had dual left sinus ostia supplying anatomically distinct left anterior descending and left circumflex arteries. No individuals with coronary arteries arising from the contralateral sinus of Valsalva were identified. Similarly, Zeppilli and colleagues [12] used two-dimensional echocardiography to screen 3,150 athletes for anomalous coronary origin, and found that only three (0.09%) had a coronary artery which originated from the incorrect aortic sinus.

Origin of either the left or right coronary artery from the contralateral sinus of Valsalva has been associated with sudden death in athletes [13,14]. Basso and colleagues reported autopsy findings from 27 young athletes who experienced sudden death during or immediately after exercise, and were found to have a coronary artery arising from the incorrect sinus of Valsalva. Origin of the left main coronary artery origin from the right sinus of Valsalva (n = 23) accounted for the majority of deaths, with only four deaths associated with origin of the right coronary artery origin from the left sinus (n = 4).

Origin of the left coronary artery from the right side can occur when the left coronary originates as a proximal branch of the right coronary artery, or when the left coronary arises from a separate ostium in the right sinus. In both anatomic variants, the left main coronary artery has several possible routes to the left side: (1) anterior to the pulmonary artery, (2) posterior to the aorta, (3) within the intraventricular septum beneath the right ventricular infundibulum, and (4) between the great vessels. The first three are generally benign and have not been associated with exercise-related death, whereas passage of the left main coronary artery between the great vessels has been associated with exercise related death [15–18].

There are two possible mechanisms for the association between a right sinus left main coronary artery and sudden death in athletes [19,20]. First, left main origin from the right sinus of Valsalva often results in an orientation of the proximal artery at an acute angle to the aortic root, making the functional ostium "slit-like" and, thus, prone to insufficient blood flow during periods of increased cardiac work. Second, if the left main coronary artery courses between the great vessels, it may be compressed by these vessels when they enlarge to accommodate the increased stroke volume of exercise. These two mechanisms are not mutually exclusive and may simultaneously contribute to myocardial ischemia.

Origin of the left main from the pulmonary trunk has only rarely been associated with exercise-related deaths. This entity was first described in 1886 and occurs in approximately one in 300,000 live births [21–23]. It is a well-recognized cause of myocardial ischemia and infarction in children, but has a mortality rate of approximately 90% by 1 year [24]. However, 10% to 15% of individuals with this anomaly remain asymptomatic during early years, ultimately survive into adulthood, and are at risk for exercise-related events. Survival into adulthood appears to require both a large dominant right coronary artery with extensive right to left collaterals, and a restricted left main coronary ostium at the site of pulmonary trunk origin to reduce the myocardial supply of deoxygenated blood [25,26]. Adults with a pulmonary arterial left main coronary artery have an estimated incidence of sudden death of 80% to 90% at a mean age of 35 years [27,28].

The diagnosis of anomalous coronary circulation in athletes is challenging and requires a high index of suspicion. This condition should be considered in young athletes presenting with symptoms of possible exercise-induced myocardial ischemia, including exertional chest discomfort, exercise intolerance, palpitations, and exercise-induced syncope. Preparticipation screening with electrocardiography and exercise stress testing cannot accurately detect these conditions [14]. Transthoracic echocardiography has been proposed for screening but has not been widely adpoted [11,12]. Conventional coronary artery angiography has long been the gold standard for the diagnosis of coronary anomalies but has been replaced by newer noninvasive imaging techniques, including coronary artery computed tomography and magnetic resonance imaging [29–32].

Athletes with an anomalous coronary anomaly associated with exercise-related sudden cardiac death should be excluded from athletic activities until the anomaly is surgically corrected [33–37].

Anomalous coronary artery course

The major coronaries and their important branches lie on the epicardial surface of the heart and provide tissue perfusion through small penetrating arterioles. Myocardial bridging refers to a segment of a major epicardial coronary artery which courses through the myocardium beneath an overlying muscular bridge. During systolic contraction, the surrounding myocardium compresses the coronary artery lumen and impedes blood flow. This entity was first recognized at autopsy in 1737, and subsequently by coronary angiography in 1960 [38,39]. The estimated prevalence of myocardial bridging ranges from 1.5% to16% in angiographic series, and as high as 80% in some autopsy reports [40,41].

The true clinical significance of myocardial bridging in the athlete is unclear. It is probable that myocardial bridging is most often benign, given the disparity between its prevalence and the incidence of related cardiac events. However, cases of exercise-induced ischemia and sudden death in the absence of other causes have been reported [7].

Several mechanisms explaining myocardial bridge related ischemia have been proposed. One possibility is that systolic epicardial coronary blood flow, of minimal significance at rest, is important at high levels of cardiac work. Reductions in total blood flow caused by systolic arterial compression could produce distal ischemia, with consequences such as malignant arrhythmias. Alternatively, myocardial bridging could accelerate local atherosclerosis or produce endovascular trauma with acute thrombus formation.

Myocardial bridging is frequent in hypertrophic cardiomyopathy [42,43]. The presence of bridging in the hypertrophic population is directly associated with the degree of septal hypertrophy and with a higher frequency of chest pain, cardiac arrest, ventricular arrhythmia, abnormal blood pressure response to exercise, and exercise induced ECG abnormalities [44]. The contribution of myocardial bridging to the well-documented risk of exercise-related cardiac events in patients with hypertrophic cardiomyopathy is uncertain.

The management of myocardial bridging in the athlete with symptoms attributable to this disorder has not been addressed in a rigorous fashion. Consensus committee guidelines, based on data derived primarily from nonathletes [45], recommend beta-blockers or calcium channel blockers for medical management to reduce heart rate and possibly to minimize the degree of intramyocardial arterial compression [46]. Intracoronary stent placement has been performed and can be considered an option in patients with symptomatic bridging that is refractory to medical interventions

[47,48]. Finally, surgical options, including dissection of the overlying myocardium and minimally invasive coronary artery bypass grafting, have been reported [49,50]. A reasonable approach to the athlete with suspected symptomatic myocardial bridging and no alternative explanatory pathology would include a stepwise escalation of therapy with periodic exercise stress testing to assess efficacy.

Secondary coronary artery pathology: acquired pathology of the coronary circulation

Atherosclerotic coronary disease

Multiple lines of evidence suggest that regular physical activity reduces the incidence of atherosclerotic coronary disease [51–54]. However, an athletic lifestyle does not completely prevent either the development of, or the adverse outcomes associated with, coronary atherosclerosis. Indeed, coronary atherosclerosis is the most frequent cause of exercise-related cardiac events in adults over the age of 30 years, but remains a rare cause of cardiac events during exercise in younger individuals [7,55,56].

There has been significant progress in our understanding of the biology and physiology of atherosclerotic coronary artery disease over the last two decades [57]. An important advance in our understanding of the atherosclerotic disease process is the recognition that acute coronary syndromes often occur in arteries without previous critical stenosis. Atherosclerotic plaque rupture and erosion in coronary segments with mild to moderate disease have been demonstrated as the inciting event leading to the acute vessel occlusion that is often responsible for myocardial infarction and subsequent sudden death.

Physical exercise may be an important stimuli for such plaque disruption [58]. Burke and colleagues [59] reported autopsy findings on 141 men with severe coronary disease, who died suddenly either at rest (n = 116) or during strenuous physical activity or emotional stress (n = 25). Culprit plaque rupture was more frequent in those individuals who died during exercise (17 out of 25, 68%) than in those who died at rest (27 out of 116, n = 23%). They concluded that acute plaque rupture is a common cause of exertional sudden death among individuals with coronary disease.

Diagnosing atherosclerotic coronary disease in athletes, and ultimately preventing exercise-related complications, is challenging. Atherosclerosis of some degree is extremely common in adults, but exercise-related cardiac events attributable to this process are comparatively rare. Exercise-related sudden death in adults occurs in only one in 15,000 to 18,000 ostensibly healthy individuals annually, although the rate of exercise-related myocardial infarction is likely higher [55,60]. Furthermore, the majority of individuals are asymptomatic before a serious or fatal event. Current consensus committee guidelines have established criteria for diagnosis, including any one of the following: (1) a history of myocardial infarction confirmed by conventional diagnostic criteria; (2) a history suggestive of angina pectoris, with objective evidence of inducible ischemia; or (3) coronary atherosclerosis of any degree demonstrated by coronary imaging studies, such as catheter-based coronary angiography, magnetic resonance angiography, or electron beam computed tomography [45].

Because an active lifestyle does not necessarily prevent atherosclerotic disease, athletes, like the general population, should be evaluated for the standard atherosclerotic risk factors, such as hypertension, diabetes, dyslipidemia, tobacco use, illicit drug use, and a family history of premature atherosclerotic disease. It is also important to inquire about exertional chest discomfort or other possible symptoms of ischemia, and to instruct adult athletes to seek medical care promptly if prodromal symptoms appear. Such complaints should not be ignored in athletes in the mistaken belief that they are immune to atherosclerotic events. All individuals with possible ischemia require diagnostic evaluation, including exercise stress testing, noninvasive imaging, or traditional coronary angiography as necessary.

Once the diagnosis of atherosclerotic coronary disease has been established, risk stratification is prudent. Current recommendations for managing of atherosclerotic disease in athletes are based primarily on data derived from nonathletes. It is likely that the risk of exercise in athletes is related to atherosclerotic disease severity, the magnitude of left ventricular dysfunction, the presence and extent of inducible ischemia, and evidence of electrical instability. Continued athletic participation is generally restricted in athletes with diagnosed atherosclerotic coronary disease, with some exceptions. Consensus recommendations for managing such patients are available [45].

Coronary artery dissection

The coronary arteries are classified as large elastic arteries. The coronary artery wall includes the intima, or inner most layer (comprised of endothelial cells), the media (made predominantly of smooth muscle), and the adventitia (consisting of extracellular matrix structural proteins and nerve fibers). These three concentric layers are tightly connected in the normal coronary artery.

Coronary artery dissection, initially described by Pretty [61] in 1931, occurs when the integrity of this trilayer structure is compromised and blood invades the vessel wall. Blood can enter the wall through a tear in the intimal layer, or via disruption of small perforator arteries that normally feed the media and the adventitia. In both variants, intramural blood compromises the vessel lumen and leads to myocardial ischemia. Coronary artery dissection can produce stable angina, acute coronary syndromes, and sudden death [62–64].

Most cases of coronary artery dissection in the present era are an iatrogenic complication of percutaneous coronary manipulation, or are due to disruption of a pre-existing atherosclerotic plaque. The term "spontaneous coronary artery dissection" is reserved for those cases without prior intravascular trauma or atherosclerosis. Spontaneous coronary artery dissection is a rare condition with an uncertain incidence rate that occurs most frequently in young women during the peripartum period or in association with oral contraceptive use [65–69]. Spontaneous coronary dissections are also observed in patients with underlying connective tissue disorders, such as Marfan's syndrome, Ehlers-Danlos syndrome, and fibromuscular dysplasia [70–72].

Physical exertion can precipitate coronary artery dissection [73–76]. The pathogenesis of exercise-induced coronary dissection is speculative, but likely results from increased shear forces caused by vigorous cardiac contraction and augmented coronary artery blood flow in individuals susceptible because of genetic variants or hormonal state.

Spontaneous coronary artery dissection should be suspected in young athletic individuals who present with clinical findings suggestive of myocardial ischemia in the absence of known atherosclerotic risk factors. This possibility should also be considered in young women with cardiac ischemia during estrogenic hormonal therapy or in the peripartum period. The possibility of coronary dissection should prompt rapid diagnostic evaluation with coronary angiography. Percutaneous coronary intervention with angioplasty and stenting has emerged as the preferred treatment strategy [77–80]. Dissection of the left main coronary artery or dissection involving multiple vessels are best managed with surgical revascularization [81,82]. Despite high rates of death associated with this condition, individuals who receive prompt treatment can survive with minimal residual morbidity [83,84]. Spontaneous dissection in athletes is rare and there are no formal recommendations regarding the management of individuals who survive their index event. Recommendations regarding further athletic participation should be considered on a case-by-case basis.

Coronary artery vasospasm

Episodic spasm of the coronary arteries with resultant myocardial ischemia, coined "variant angina," was described in 1959 by Prinzmetal and colleagues [85]. This phenomenon occurs most frequently at rest and is usually not precipitated by emotional stress or physical exertion. The clinical manifestations of this disorder include typical chest pain with ST-segment elevation on the 12-lead electrocardiogram that are indistinguishable from those associated with acute thrombotic occlusion of a coronary artery, except that the ST elevation with vasospasm is promptly reversible. Coronary vasospasm appears to occur most frequently in regions of the coronary circulation with pre-existing atherosclerotic disease, with or without true luminal narrowing [86,87]. The mediating mechanisms are incompletely defined, but probably include reduced production of local vasodilatory factors because of atherosclerotic endothelial damage or a systemic alteration in vasomotor control [88–90].

Classic variant angina occurs at rest, but exercise can trigger attacks in some individuals. Yasue and colleagues [91] reported experience with 13 individuals with this condition who had symptoms that occurred during exercise treadmill testing. In all individuals attacks were provoked during morning physical exertion but did not occur during repeat afternoon testing. This suggestion of an interaction between variant angina attacks and circadian rhythm has been observed by other investigators [92]. Exercise has also been documented to produce paradoxical coronary vasoconstriction in individuals with underlying atherosclerotic disease. The normal coronary arteries vasodilate during exercise but may constrict during exercise if there is underlying, even minimal, atherosclerosis [93]. The contribution

of vasospasm to acute exercise-related cardiac events has never been well documented, but may account for some sudden deaths or acute myocardial infarctions in the absence of "important" atherosclerosis by angiography or necropsy. These examinations, however, cannot exclude more frequent scenarios, such as a thrombotic event with subsequent clot resolution.

Coronary vasospasm should be suspected in athletic individuals who develop typical chest pain, either at rest or during physical exertion, and who have no evidence of flow obstructing atherosclerotic disease during diagnostic testing. Exercise stress testing has limited sensitivity for the detection of this condition. Coronary angiography and ventriculography performed during an episode of variant angina typically demonstrates proximal coronary artery narrowing or occlusion, with resultant abnormalities in left ventricular function. Both spasm and consequent myocardial dysfunction are eliminated by the introduction of systemic or intracoronary nitroglycerin, or an alternative vasodilator. Spasm appears to occur most frequently in the right coronary artery, followed by involvement of the left anterior descending artery [94]. Provocative testing during angiography with ergonovine and related agents is rarely performed, but guidelines for this strategy have been developed [95].

Most individuals with this condition follow a benign clinical course, though—rarely—vasospasm can precipitate serious complications of myocardial ischemia, including infarction, arrhythmia, or sudden death [96]. Pharmacologic intervention with calcium channel blockers and long acting nitrates is effective [97,98]. Athletes with documented vasospasm should also undergo atherosclerosis risk factor management because underlying atherosclerosis contributes to abnormal coronary vasomotion. The risk of vigorous exercise in athletes associated with vasospastic angina is unknown. Recommendations for athletic activity should be based on evidence that exercise produces vasospasm in the athlete, the ability to control symptoms with medications, and the presence of underlying atherosclerosis. Consensus guidelines favor marked restriction of physical activity in these athletes.

Summary

The physical demands on athletic participants require high levels of myocardial function. The augmentation of myocardial function that accompanies vigorous exercise is dependent upon adequate coronary artery blood flow reserve. Coronary artery pathology can limit coronary blood flow and produce exertional myocardial ischemia with its clinical consequences. The clinician charged with the care of athletes must have a high index of suspicion for underlying coronary artery pathology when faced with an individual with suggestive symptoms. Management includes treatment of the underlying coronary condition and restriction of athletic participation when appropriate.

References

[1] Reese DE, Mikawa T, Bader DM. Development of the coronary vessel system. Circ Res 2002;91(9): 761–8.

[2] Mikawa T, Gourdie RG. Pericardial mesoderm generates a population of coronary smooth muscle cells migrating into the heart along with ingrowth of the epicardial organ. Dev Biol 1996;174(2):221–32.

[3] Chilian WM. Coronary microcirculation in health and disease. Summary of an NHLBI workshop. Circulation 1997;95(2):522–8.

[4] Yada T, Richmond KN, Van Bibber R, et al. Role of adenosine in local metabolic coronary vasodilation. Am J Physiol 1999;276(5 Pt 2):H1425–33.

[5] Feigl EO. Neural control of coronary blood flow. J Vasc Res 1998;35(2):85–92.

[6] Maron BJ, Epstein SE, Roberts WC. Causes of sudden death in competitive athletes. J Am Coll Cardiol 1986;7(1):204–14.

[7] Maron BJ, Shirani J, Poliac LC, et al. Sudden death in young competitive athletes. Clinical, demographic, and pathological profiles. JAMA 1996; 276(3):199–204.

[8] Corrado D, Thiene G, Nava A, et al. Sudden death in young competitive athletes: clinicopathologic correlations in 22 cases. Am J Med 1990;89(5):588–96.

[9] Roberts WC. Major anomalies of coronary arterial origin seen in adulthood. Am Heart J 1986;111(5): 941–63.

[10] Harikrishnan S, Jacob SP, Tharakan J, et al. Congenital coronary anomalies of origin and distribution in adults: a coronary arteriographic study. Indian Heart J 2002;54(3):271–5.

[11] Pelliccia A, Spataro A, Maron BJ. Prospective echocardiographic screening for coronary artery anomalies in 1,360 elite competitive athletes. Am J Cardiol 1993;72(12):978–9.

[12] Zeppilli P, dello Russo A, Santini C, et al. In vivo detection of coronary artery anomalies in asymptomatic athletes by echocardiographic screening. Chest 1998;114(1):89–93.

[13] Frescura C, Basso C, Thiene G, et al. Anomalous origin of coronary arteries and risk of sudden death: a study based on an autopsy population of congenital heart disease. Hum Pathol 1998;29(7):689–95.

[14] Basso C, Maron BJ, Corrado D, et al. Clinical profile of congenital coronary artery anomalies with origin from the wrong aortic sinus leading to sudden death in young competitive athletes. J Am Coll Cardiol 2000;35(6):1493–501.

[15] Cheitlin MD, De Castro CM, McAllister HA. Sudden death as a complication of anomalous left coronary origin from the anterior sinus of Valsalva, a not-so-minor congenital anomaly. Circulation 1974;50(4):780–7.

[16] Benson PA. Anomalous aortic origin of coronary artery with sudden death: case report and review. Am Heart J 1970;79(2):254–7.

[17] Taylor AJ, Rogan KM, Virmani R. Sudden cardiac death associated with isolated congenital coronary artery anomalies. J Am Coll Cardiol 1992;20(3): 640–7.

[18] Roberts WC, Shirani J. The four subtypes of anomalous origin of the left main coronary artery from the right aortic sinus (or from the right coronary artery). Am J Cardiol 1992;70(1):119–21.

[19] Barth CW 3rd, Roberts WC. Left main coronary artery originating from the right sinus of Valsalva and coursing between the aorta and pulmonary trunk. J Am Coll Cardiol 1986;7(2):366–73.

[20] Davia JE, Green DC, Cheitlin MD, et al. Anomalous left coronary artery origin from the right coronary sinus. Am Heart J 1984;108(1):165–6.

[21] Keith JD. The anomalous origin of the left coronary artery from the pulmonary artery. Br Heart J 1959; 21(2):149–61.

[22] Backer CL, Stout MJ, Zales VR, et al. Anomalous origin of the left coronary artery. A twenty-year review of surgical management. J Thorac Cardiovasc Surg 1992;103(6):1049–57 [discussion: 1048–57].

[23] Brooks S. Two cases of abnormal coronary artery of the heart arising from the pulmonary artery: with some remarks upon the effect of this anomaly in producing cirsoid dilation of the vessels. J Anat Physiol 1886;20:26–32.

[24] Wesselhoeft H, Fawcett JS, Johnson AL. Anomalous origin of the left coronary artery from the pulmonary trunk. Its clinical spectrum, pathology, and pathophysiology, based on a review of 140 cases with seven further cases. Circulation 1968;38(2): 403–25.

[25] Berdjis F, Takahashi M, Wells WJ, et al. Anomalous left coronary artery from the pulmonary artery. Significance of intercoronary collaterals. J Thorac Cardiovasc Surg 1994;108(1):17–20.

[26] Smith A, Arnold R, Anderson RH, et al. Anomalous origin of the left coronary artery from the pulmonary trunk. Anatomic findings in relation to pathophysiology and surgical repair. J Thorac Cardiovasc Surg 1989;98(1):16–24.

[27] Alexi-Meskishvili V, Berger F, Weng Y, et al. Anomalous origin of the left coronary artery from the pulmonary artery in adults. J Card Surg 1995;10(4 Pt 1): 309–15.

[28] Fernandes ED, Kadivar H, Hallman GL, et al. Congenital malformations of the coronary arteries: the Texas Heart Institute experience. Ann Thorac Surg 1992;54(4):732–40.

[29] Memisoglu E, Ropers D, Hobikoglu G, et al. Usefulness of electron beam computed tomography for diagnosis of an anomalous origin of a coronary artery from the opposite sinus. Am J Cardiol 2005;96(10):1452–5.

[30] Taylor AM, Thorne SA, Rubens MB, et al. Coronary artery imaging in grown up congenital heart disease: complementary role of magnetic resonance and x-ray coronary angiography. Circulation 2000; 101(14):1670–8.

[31] McConnell MV, Ganz P, Selwyn AP, et al. Identification of anomalous coronary arteries and their anatomic course by magnetic resonance coronary angiography. Circulation 1995;92(11):3158–62.

[32] Memisoglu E, Hobikoglu G, Tepe MS, et al. Congenital coronary anomalies in adults: comparison of anatomic course visualization by catheter angiography and electron beam CT. Catheter Cardiovasc Interv 2005;66(1):34–42.

[33] Maron BJ, Isner JM, McKenna WJ. 26th Bethesda conference: recommendations for determining eligibility for competition in athletes with cardiovascular abnormalities. Task Force 3: hypertrophic cardiomyopathy, myocarditis and other myopericardial diseases and mitral valve prolapse. J Am Coll Cardiol 1994;24(4):880–5.

[34] Thomas D, Salloum J, Montalescot G, et al. Anomalous coronary arteries coursing between the aorta and pulmonary trunk: clinical indications for coronary artery bypass. Eur Heart J 1991;12(7):832–4.

[35] Laks H, Ardehali A, Grant PW, et al. Aortic implantation of anomalous left coronary artery. An improved surgical approach. J Thorac Cardiovasc Surg 1995;109(3):519–23.

[36] Lambert V, Touchot A, Losay J, et al. Midterm results after surgical repair of the anomalous origin of the coronary artery. Circulation 1996;94(9 Suppl): II38–43.

[37] Erez E, Tam VK, Doublin NA, et al. Anomalous coronary artery with aortic origin and course between the great arteries: improved diagnosis, anatomic findings, and surgical treatment. Ann Thorac Surg 2006;82(3):973–7.

[38] Reyman H. Disertatio de vasis cordis propriis. Göttingen: Med Diss. Univ Göttingen 1737;1–32.

[39] Portmann W, Iwig J. [The intramural coronary on the angiogram]. Die intramurale koronarie im angiogramm. Fortschritte Auf Dem Gebiete Der Ronteenstrahlen 1960;92:129–32.

[40] Rossi L, Dander B, Nidasio GP, et al. Myocardial bridges and ischemic heart disease. Eur Heart J 1980;1(4):239–45.

[41] Geirenger E. The mural coronary. Am Heart J 1951; 41:359–68.

[42] Mohiddin SA, Begley D, Shih J, et al. Myocardial bridging does not predict sudden death in children with hypertrophic cardiomyopathy but is associated with more severe cardiac disease. J Am Coll Cardiol 2000;36(7):2270–8.

[43] Sorajja P, Ommen SR, Nishimura RA, et al. Myocardial bridging in adult patients with hypertrophic cardiomyopathy. J Am Coll Cardiol 2003;42(5): 889–94.

[44] Yetman AT, McCrindle BW, MacDonald C, et al. Myocardial bridging in children with hypertrophic cardiomyopathy—a risk factor for sudden death. N Engl J Med 1998;339(17):1201–9.

[45] Thompson PD, Balady GJ, Chaitman BR, et al. Task Force 6: coronary artery disease. J Am Coll Cardiol 2005;45(8):1348–53.

[46] Schwarz ER, Klues HG, vom Dahl J, et al. Functional, angiographic and intracoronary Doppler flow characteristics in symptomatic patients with myocardial bridging: effect of short-term intravenous beta-blocker medication. J Am Coll Cardiol 1996;27(7):1637–45.

[47] Klues HG, Schwarz ER, vom Dahl J, et al. Disturbed intracoronary hemodynamics in myocardial bridging: early normalization by intracoronary stent placement. Circulation 1997;96(9):2905–13.

[48] Haager PK, Schwarz ER, vom Dahl J, et al. Long term angiographic and clinical follow up in patients with stent implantation for symptomatic myocardial bridging. Heart 2000;84(4):403–8.

[49] Iversen S, Hake U, Mayer E, et al. Surgical treatment of myocardial bridging causing coronary artery obstruction. Scand J Thorac Cardiovasc Surg 1992;26(2):107–11.

[50] Pratt JW, Michler RE, Pala J, et al. Minimally invasive coronary artery bypass grafting for myocardial muscle bridging. Heart Surg Forum 1999;2(3): 250–3.

[51] Leon AS, Connett J, Jacobs DR Jr, et al. Leisuretime physical activity levels and risk of coronary heart disease and death. The Multiple Risk Factor Intervention Trial. JAMA 1987;258(17): 2388–95.

[52] Blair SN, Kohl HW 3rd, Paffenbarger RS Jr, et al. Physical fitness and all-cause mortality. A prospective study of healthy men and women. JAMA 1989;262(17):2395–401.

[53] Kannel WB, Wilson P, Blair SN. Epidemiological assessment of the role of physical activity and fitness in development of cardiovascular disease. Am Heart J 1985;109(4):876–85.

[54] Pomrehn PR, Wallace RB, Burmeister LF. Ischemic heart disease mortality in Iowa farmers. The influence of life-style. JAMA 1982;248(9):1073–6.

[55] Thompson PD, Funk EJ, Carleton RA, et al. Incidence of death during jogging in Rhode Island from 1975 through 1980. JAMA 1982;247(18):2535–8.

[56] Van Camp SP, Bloor CM, Mueller FO, et al. Non-traumatic sports death in high school and college athletes. Med Sci Sports Exerc 1995;27(5):641–7.

[57] Virmani R, Burke AP, Farb A, et al. Pathology of the vulnerable plaque. J Am Coll Cardiol 2006; 47(8 Suppl):C13–8.

[58] Black A, Black MM, Gensini G. Exertion and acute coronary artery injury. Angiology 1975;26(11): 759–83.

[59] Burke AP, Farb A, Malcom GT, et al. Plaque rupture and sudden death related to exertion in men with coronary artery disease. JAMA 1999;281(10):921–6.

[60] Siscovick DS, Weiss NS, Fletcher RH, et al. The incidence of primary cardiac arrest during vigorous exercise. N Engl J Med 1984;311(14):874–7.

[61] Pretty HC. Dissecting aneurysm of coronary artery in a woman aged 42: rupture. BMJ 1931;1:667.

[62] DeMaio SJ Jr, Kinsella SH, Silverman ME. Clinical course and long-term prognosis of spontaneous coronary artery dissection. Am J Cardiol 1989;64(8): 471–4.

[63] Basso C, Morgagni GL, Thiene G. Spontaneous coronary artery dissection: a neglected cause of acute myocardial ischaemia and sudden death. Heart 1996;75(5):451–4.

[64] Jorgensen MB, Aharonian V, Mansukhani P, et al. Spontaneous coronary dissection: a cluster of cases with this rare finding. Am Heart J 1994;127(5): 1382–7.

[65] Frey BW, Grant RJ. Pregnancy-associated coronary artery dissection: a case report. J Emerg Med 2006; 30(3):307–10.

[66] Klutstein MW, Tzivoni D, Bitran D, et al. Treatment of spontaneous coronary artery dissection: report of three cases. Cathet Cardiovasc Diagn 1997; 40(4):372–6.

[67] Koul AK, Hollander G, Moskovits N, et al. Coronary artery dissection during pregnancy and the postpartum period: two case reports and review of literature. Catheter Cardiovasc Interv 2001;52(1): 88–94.

[68] Azam MN, Roberts DH, Logan WF. Spontaneous coronary artery dissection associated with oral contraceptive use. Int J Cardiol 1995;48(2):195–8.

[69] Heefner WA. Dissecting hematoma of the coronary artery. A possible complication of oral contraceptive therapy. JAMA 1973;223(5):550–1.

[70] Lie JT, Berg KK. Isolated fibromuscular dysplasia of the coronary arteries with spontaneous dissection and myocardial infarction. Hum Pathol 1987;18(6): 654–6.

[71] Catanese V, Venot P, Lemesle F, et al. [Myocardial infarction by spontaneous dissection of coronary arteries in a subject with type IV Ehlers-Danlos syndrome]. Presse Med 1995;24(29):1345–7 [in French].

[72] Angiolillo DJ, Moreno R, Macaya C. Isolated distal coronary dissection in Marfan syndrome. Ital Heart J 2004;5(4):305–6.

[73] Nalbandian RM, Chason JL. Intramural (intramedial) dissecting hematomas in normal or otherwise unremarkable coronary arteries. A "rare" cause of death. Am J Clin Pathol 1965;43:348–56.

[74] Giri S, Thompson PD, Kiernan FJ, et al. Clinical and angiographic characteristics of exertion-related acute myocardial infarction. JAMA 1999;282(18): 1731–6.

[75] Ellis CJ, Haywood GA, Monro JL. Spontaneous coronary artery dissection in a young woman resulting from an intense gymnasium "work-out". Int J Cardiol 1994;47(2):193–4.

[76] Sherrid MV, Mieres J, Mogtader A, et al. Onset during exercise of spontaneous coronary artery dissection and sudden death. Occurrence in a trained athlete: case report and review of prior cases. Chest 1995;108(1):284–7.

[77] Cheung S, Mithani V, Watson RM. Healing of spontaneous coronary dissection in the context of glycoprotein IIB/IIIA inhibitor therapy: a case report. Catheter Cardiovasc Interv 2000;51(1):95–100.

[78] Hong MK, Satler LF, Mintz GS, et al. Treatment of spontaneous coronary artery dissection with intracoronary stenting. Am Heart J 1996;132(1 Pt 1): 200–2.

[79] Hanratty CG, McKeown PP, O'Keeffe DB. Coronary stenting in the setting of spontaneous coronary artery dissection. Int J Cardiol 1998;67(3):197–9.

[80] Leclerc KM, Mascette AM, Schachter DT, et al. Spontaneous coronary artery dissection in a young woman treated with extensive coronary stenting. J Invasive Cardiol 1999;11(4):237–41.

[81] Boyd WD, Walley VM, Keon WJ. Surgical treatment of spontaneous left main coronary artery dissection. Ann Thorac Surg 1988;46(4):483.

[82] Atay Y, Yagdi T, Turkoglu C, et al. Spontaneous dissection of the left main coronary artery: a case report and review of the literature. J Card Surg 1996; 11(5):371–5.

[83] Zampieri P, Aggio S, Roncon L, et al. Follow up after spontaneous coronary artery dissection: a report of five cases. Heart 1996;75(2):206–9.

[84] Longheval G, Badot V, Cosyns B, et al. Spontaneous coronary artery dissection: favorable outcome illustrated by angiographic data. Clin Cardiol 1999; 22(5):374–5.

[85] Prinzmetal M, Kennamer R, Merliss R, et al. Angina pectoris. I. A variant form of angina pectoris; preliminary report. Am J Med 1959;27:375–88.

[86] Gordon JB, Ganz P, Nabel EG, et al. Atherosclerosis influences the vasomotor response of epicardial coronary arteries to exercise. J Clin Invest 1989; 83(6):1946–52.

[87] Mark DB, Califf RM, Morris KG, et al. Clinical characteristics and long-term survival of patients with variant angina. Circulation 1984;69(5):880–8.

[88] Cox ID, Kaski JC, Clague JR. Endothelial dysfunction in the absence of coronary atheroma causing Prinzmetal's angina. Heart 1997;77(6):584.

[89] Hamabe A, Takase B, Uehata A, et al. Impaired en-
dothelium-dependent vasodilation in the brachial
artery in variant angina pectoris and the effect of
intravenous administration of vitamin C. Am J Cardiol 2001;87(10):1154–9.

[90] Sakata Y, Komamura K, Hirayama A, et al. Elevation of the plasma histamine concentration in the
coronary circulation in patients with variant angina.
Am J Cardiol 1996;77(12):1121–6.

[91] Yasue H, Omote S, Takizawa A, et al. Circadian
variation of exercise capacity in patients with Prinzmetal's variant angina: role of exercise-induced coronary
arterial spasm. Circulation 1979;59(5):938–48.

[92] Ogawa H, Yasue H, Oshima S, et al. Circadian variation of plasma fibrinopeptide A level in patients
with variant angina. Circulation 1989;80(6):1617–26.

[93] Nabel EG, Ganz P, Gordon JB, et al. Dilation of
normal and constriction of atherosclerotic coronary
arteries caused by the cold pressor test. Circulation
1988;77(1):43–52.

[94] Pepine CJ, el-Tamimi H, Lambert CR. Prinzmetal's angina (variant angina). Heart Dis Stroke 1992;1(5):281–6.

[95] Gibbons RJ, Abrams J, Chatterjee K, et al. ACC/
AHA 2002 guideline update for the management
of patients with chronic stable angina—summary article: a report of the American College of Cardiol-
ogy/American Heart Association Task Force on
practice guidelines (Committee on the Management
of Patients With Chronic Stable Angina). J Am Coll
Cardiol 2003;41(1):159–68.

[96] Bory M, Pierron F, Panagides D, et al. Coronary artery spasm in patients with normal or near normal
coronary arteries. Long-term follow-up of 277
patients. Eur Heart J 1996;17(7):1015–21.

[97] Antman E, Muller J, Goldberg S, et al. Nifedipine
therapy for coronary-artery spasm. Experience
in 127 patients. N Engl J Med 1980;302(23):
1269–73.

[98] Lombardi M, Morales MA, Michelassi C, et al.
Efficacy of isosorbide-5-mononitrate versus nifedipine in preventing spontaneous and ergonovine-
induced myocardial ischaemia. A double-blind,
placebo-controlled study. Eur Heart J 1993;14(6):
845–51.

CARDIOLOGY
CLINICS

Cardiol Clin 25 (2007) 441–448

Athletes with Systemic Hypertension

Robert H. Fagard, MD, PhD

Hypertension and Cardiovascular Rehabilitation Unit, Department of Cardiovascular Diseases, University of Leuven,
KU Leuven, U.Z. Gasthuisberg – Hypertensie, Herestraat 49, B-3000 Leuven, Belgium

Epidemiology

Blood pressure increases with age. Systolic blood pressure continues to increase throughout adult life, related to progressive arterial stiffening, whereas diastolic blood pressure plateaus in the sixth decade of life and decreases thereafter [1]. Blood pressure is lower in women than in men below the age of about 50, rises more steeply in women around menopause, and becomes higher in women than in men thereafter.

In recent epidemiologic studies, hypertension is defined as systolic blood pressure greater than or equal to 140 mm Hg or diastolic blood pressure greater than or equal to 90 mm Hg, or being on antihypertensive treatment. The prevalence of hypertension in the population amounts to about 25% and is expected to increase to up to about 29% in 2025 [2].

When broken down by age and gender, the prevalence is approximately 15%, 30%, and 55% in men aged 18 to 39, 40 to 59, and 60 and older, respectively, and about 5%, 30%, and 65% in women in these age groups. The prevalence of isolated systolic hypertension is very low before the age of 50, but increases sharply thereafter. These epidemiologic data indicate that hypertension may already be present in the young athlete, although rarely, but occurs more frequently in the older sportsman.

Unless blood pressure is measured, hypertension may remain undetected because it usually causes no symptoms. However, about 25% of patients who have hypertension by conventional measurements have a normal blood pressure on 24-hour ambulatory monitoring or on home blood pressure measurements; this phenomenon is the so-called "white-coat" or isolated clinic hypertension [3,4]. Young athletes with clinic hypertension often have normal blood pressure on ambulatory monitoring [5]. On the other hand, patients may have masked or isolated ambulatory hypertension, which is characterized by a normal blood pressure in the office and an elevated blood pressure out of the office [6].

Hypertension as a cardiovascular risk factor

Hypertension is associated with an increased incidence of all-cause and cardiovascular mortality, sudden death, stroke, coronary heart disease, heart failure, atrial fibrillation, peripheral arterial disease, and renal insufficiency. In the population at large, the relationship between cardiovascular complications and blood pressure is linear [7]. The prognosis of white-coat hypertension is better than that of sustained ambulatory hypertension, and studies suggest that it is even similar to that of persons with true normal blood pressure, whereas patients who have masked hypertension appear to have a worse outcome than true normotensives [3,4,6,8–10].

Despite conclusive evidence that antihypertensive therapy reduces the complications of hypertension [1,11], only about one half of all patients who have hypertension are under treatment and only a fraction of these have normal blood pressure [12,13]. Systolic blood pressure appears to be more difficult to control than diastolic blood pressure, particularly in older patients.

Classification of hypertension

The classification of hypertension is based on multiple conventional blood pressure measurements taken on separate occasions, in the sitting

E-mail address: robert.fagard@uz.kuleuven.ac.be

doi:10.1016/j.ccl.2007.07.001

cardiology.theclinics.com

position, by use of a mercury sphygmomanometer or another calibrated device. Table 1 summarizes the definitions and classification of blood pressure levels, according to the European Society of Hypertension – European Society of Cardiology guidelines for the management of arterial hypertension [1,14]. The universally accepted blood pressure threshold for hypertension is 140/90 mm Hg.

Twenty-four hour ambulatory blood pressure monitoring should be considered in cases of suspected white-coat hypertension, considerable variability of office blood pressure, marked discrepancy between blood pressure measured in the office and at home, and in subjects with high office blood pressure and low global cardiovascular risk. The threshold for the definition of hypertension is 130/80 mm Hg for 24-hour blood pressure. The threshold for daytime ambulatory blood pressure and the self-measured blood pressure at home is 135/85 mm Hg. Patients above the threshold for conventional blood pressure and below the threshold for the out-of-office pressure are considered to have white-coat or isolated office hypertension and the reverse is true for masked or isolated ambulatory hypertension [1,15].

Approximately 95% of patients who have hypertension have essential or primary hypertension, which results from an interaction between genetic factors and lifestyle/environmental factors that include being overweight, high salt intake, excessive alcohol consumption, and physical inactivity. The main causes of secondary hypertension involve renovascular, renal, and adrenal abnormalities [1].

The role of ergogenic aids in increasing blood pressure should be considered in the hypertensive sportsman or athlete. Athletes may abuse prohibited substances such as anabolic steroids, erythropoietin, stimulants, and so forth. The uncontrolled use of these agents has been associated with numerous side effects, including hypertension. Also, the use of nonsteroidal anti-inflammatory drugs should be specifically considered because these compounds may increase blood pressure and are commonly used in the athletic setting [16].

Assessment of the severity of hypertension and risk stratification

The severity of hypertension depends not only on the blood pressure level (see Table 1) but also on the presence of other cardiovascular risk factors, target organ damage, and cardiovascular and renal complications. Table 2 summarizes the classification based on the overall cardiovascular risk [1,14]. The terms low, moderate, high, and very high added risk, in comparison with healthy normotensives without risk factors, are calibrated to indicate an approximate absolute 10-year risk of cardiovascular disease of less than 15%, 15% to 20%, 20% to 30% and greater than 30%, respectively, according to the Framingham criteria, or an approximate absolute risk of fatal cardiovascular disease of less than 4%, 4% to 5%, 6% to 8% and more than 8%, according to the European SCORE system [17].

The risk stratification is based on the accumulated number of selected risk factors, the presence of target organ damage, or cardiovascular or renal disease, as outlined in Table 2. With regard to left ventricular hypertrophy, it should be noted that sports activity itself may induce hypertrophy; the extent and distribution of hypertrophy and assessment of diastolic left ventricular function may help to distinguish between hypertensive heart disease and athlete's heart [18–21]. Athlete's heart typically shows normal diastolic filling and relaxation, and is considered a physiologic adaptation to training, in contrast to the hypertrophy secondary to hypertension. Hypertensive patients usually have concentric left ventricular hypertrophy (but eccentric hypertrophy has also been described) [22]; whether or not hypertension in an athlete will accentuate the development and extent of left ventricular hypertrophy, or whether athletic conditioning in a hypertensive patient will worsen the left ventricular hypertrophy, is not known.

The importance of the risk stratification is that hypertensive patients at high or very high added risk should be treated promptly with

Table 1

Definitions and classification of clinic blood pressure levels (mm Hg)

Category	Systolic		Diastolic
Optimal	<120	and/or	<80
Normal	120–129	and/or	80–84
High normal	130–139	and/or	85–89
Grade 1 hypertension	140–159	and/or	90–99
Grade 2 hypertension	160–179	and/or	100–109
Grade 3 hypertension	≥180	and/or	≥110
Isolated systolic hypertension	≥140	and/or	<90

Isolated systolic hypertension can also be graded (grades 1, 2, 3) according to systolic blood pressure values in the ranges indicated, provided diastolic values are less than 90 mm Hg.

Table 2
Stratification of cardiovascular risk in four categories

Other risk factors, target organ damage, or disease	Blood pressure (mm Hg)				
	Normal (SBP 120–129 or DBP 80–84)	High normal (SBP 130–139 or DBP 85–89)	Grade 1 HT (SBP 140–159 or DBP 90–99)	Grade 2 HT (SBP 160–179 or DBP 100–109)	Grade 3 HT (SBP ≥ 180 or DBP ≥ 110)
No other risk factors[a]	Average risk	Average risk	Low added risk	Moderate added risk	High added risk
1–2 risk factors[a]	Low added risk	Low added risk	Moderate added risk	Moderate added risk	Very high added risk
3 or more risk factors[a], TOD[b], MS or diabetes	Moderate added risk	High added risk	High added risk	High added risk	Very high added risk
Established CV or renal disease[c]	Very high added risk	Very high added risk	Very high added risk	Very high added risk	Very high added risk

Low, moderate, high and very high added risk indicate an approximate 10-year risk of fatal or nonfatal cardiovascular disease of less than 15%, 15% to 20%, 20% to 30%, and higher than 30%, respectively; or a risk of fatal cardiovascular disease of less than 4%, 4% to 5%, 5% to 8%, and higher than 8%, according to SCORE charts.

Abbreviations: CV, cardiovascular; DBP, diastolic blood pressure; HT, hypertension; SBP, systolic blood pressure; MS, metabolic syndrome; TOD, target organ damage.

[a] Risk factors used for stratification are blood pressure level; levels of pulse pressure (in the elderly); gender and age (men > 55 years; women > 65 years); smoking; dyslipidemia (total cholesterol > 190 mg/dL or low-density lipoprotein cholesterol > 115 mg/dL, or high-density lipoprotein cholesterol < 40 mg/dL in men and < 46 mg/dL in women, or triglycerides > 150 mg/dL); abdominal obesity (men ≥ 102 cm; women ≥ 88 cm); first-degree family history of premature cardiovascular disease (men < 55 years; women < 65 years); fasting plasma glucose (102–125 mg/dL); abnormal glucose tolerance test.

[b] Target organ damage includes hypertension-induced left ventricular hypertrophy; ultrasound evidence of arterial wall thickening or atherosclerotic plaque; slight increase in plasma creatinine (men 1.3–1.5 mg/dL; women 1.2–1.4 mg/dL); estimated glomerular filtration rate < 60 mL/min/1.73 m^2); presence of microalbuminuria; carotid-femoral pulse wave velocity > 12 m/s; ankle/brachial blood pressure ratio < 0.9.

[c] Diseases include cerebrovascular disease (stroke; transient ischemic attack); ischemic heart disease (myocardial infarction, angina, coronary revascularisation); heart failure; peripheral vascular disease; renal disease (diabetic nephropathy; renal impairment; proteinuria); advanced retinopathy (hemorrhages; exudates; papiledema).

antihypertensive drugs, whereas patients at low or moderate added risk are only treated when hypertension persists despite lifestyle measures. An alternative way to estimate risk in those who are not at high or very high added risk according to Table 2 is to use the European SCORE system [17].

Assessment of the risk associated with exercise

Exercise-related sudden death at a younger age is mainly attributed to hypertrophic cardiomyopathy, anomalies of the coronary arteries, or arrhythmogenic right ventricular dysplasia [21,23–25], and is unlikely to be related to hypertension. On the other hand, coronary heart disease has been identified in approximately 75% of victims of exercise-related sudden death above the age of 35 [26]. Whether or not high blood pressure is a cause of exercise-related sudden death on its own is not known, but hypertension is certainly

a major risk factor for the development of coronary artery disease. In addition, hypertension-induced left ventricular hypertrophy may cause life-threatening ventricular arrhythmias [27]. It is likely that the risk associated with exercise can be derived from the overall risk stratification (see Table 2). Therefore, the general approach to the hypertensive patient should also apply to the exercising patient.

Diagnostic evaluation

Diagnostic procedures are aimed at

Establishing blood pressure levels
Identifying secondary causes of hypertension
Evaluating the overall cardiovascular risk by searching for other risk factors, target organ damage and concomitant diseases, or accompanying clinical conditions [1,14].

Diagnostic procedures comprise a thorough individual and family history; physical examination, including repeated blood pressure measurements according to established recommendations; and laboratory and instrumental investigations, of which some should be considered part of the routine approach in all subjects with high blood pressure, some are recommended, and some are indicated only when suggested by the core examinations.

Routine tests include hemoglobin and hematocrit; serum potassium, creatinine and uric acid; estimated glomerular filtration rate; fasting plasma glucose; serum total, low-density and high-density lipoprotein cholesterol, and triglycerides; urine analysis complemented by microalbuminuria dipstick test and sediment examination; and standard electrocardiography. In addition, in the competitive athlete with hypertension, echocardiography and exercise testing with electrocardiography and blood pressure monitoring are indicated as routine tests [28,29].

Recommended tests include echocardiography; carotid ultrasound; pulse wave velocity measurement; ankle-brachial blood pressure ratio index; fundoscopy; quantitative proteinuria (if dipstick test positive); or glucose tolerance test (if fasting plasma glucose > 100 mg/dL); and home and 24-hour blood pressure monitoring. Extended evaluation may be necessary, based on the findings from these investigations [1,14].

The indication for exercise testing depends on the patient's risk profile and on the amateur/leisure-time sports characteristics (Table 3) [29,30]. In patients who have hypertension and are about to engage in intense (although amateur) exercise training (ie, intensity ≥60% of maximum), a medically supervised peak or symptom-limited exercise test with electrocardiography (or cardiopulmonary testing) and blood pressure monitoring is warranted. In asymptomatic men or women with low or moderate added risk (see Table 2) who engage in low-to-moderate leisure-time physical activity (ie, intensity <60% of maximum), further testing beyond the routine evaluation is generally not needed. Asymptomatic patients with high or very high added risk may benefit from exercise testing before engaging in moderate-intensity exercise (ie, 40%-60% of maximum). Patients who have exertional dyspnea, chest discomfort, or palpitations need further examination, which includes exercise testing, echocardiography, Holter monitoring, or combinations thereof.

A major problem with exercise testing in a population with a low probability of coronary heart disease and in subjects with left ventricular hypertrophy is that most positive tests on electrocardiography are falsely positive. Stress myocardial scintigraphy or echocardiography, and, ultimately, coronaroangiography, may be indicated in cases of doubt. Evidence is inconclusive that blood pressure response to exercise, in addition to blood pressure at rest, should play a role in the recommendations for exercise [31]; however, subjects with an excessive rise of blood pressure during exercise are more prone to develop hypertension and should be followed up more closely [29]. Finally, physicians should be aware that high blood pressure may impair exercise tolerance [32].

Effects of exercise on blood pressure

Dynamic exercise

Blood pressure increases during acute dynamic exercise in proportion to the intensity of the effort [32]. During long-term, steady-state exercise, blood pressure tends to decrease after an initial increase of short duration. The increase is greater for systolic than for diastolic blood pressure, which increases only slightly or even remains unchanged. For the same oxygen consumption, the rise is more pronounced in older subjects and when exercise is performed with smaller versus larger muscle groups. The exercise is usually followed by postexercise hypotension, which may last for several hours and is generally more pronounced and of longer duration in patients who have hypertension than in normotensive subjects [30].

Table 3
Indications for exercise testing for sports participation in patients who have hypertension

Demands of exercise (static or dynamic)	Risk category	
	Low or moderate	High or very high[a]
Light (<40% of max)	No	No
Moderate (40%-59% of max)	No	Yes
High (≥60% of max)	Yes	Yes

[a] In case of an associated clinical condition, the recommendations for the specific condition should be observed.

Cross-sectional and longitudinal epidemiologic studies indicate that physical inactivity and low fitness levels are associated with higher blood pressure levels and increased incidence of hypertension in the population [33]. Meta-analyses of randomized, controlled intervention studies concluded that regular dynamic endurance training at moderate intensity significantly reduces blood pressure [34–36].

A recent meta-analysis involved 72 trials and 105 study groups [36]. After weighting for the number of participants, training was responsible for a significant net reduction of resting and daytime ambulatory blood pressure (3.0/2.4 mm Hg and 3.3/3.5 mm Hg, respectively). The reduction of resting blood pressure was more pronounced in the 30 hypertensive study groups (−6.9/−4.9) than in the others (−1.9/−1.6). Evidence was not convincing that the degree of reduction in blood pressure was related to the intensity of exercise training, when this ranged between about 40% and 80% of maximal aerobic power [34]. Systemic vascular resistance decreased by 7.1%, plasma norepinephrine by 29%, and plasma renin activity by 20%. Body weight decreased by 1.2 kg, waist circumference by 2.8 cm, percent body fat by 1.4%, and the homeostatic model assessment (HOMA) index of insulin resistance by 0.31 units; high-density lipoprotein cholesterol increased by 0.032 mg/dL. Therefore, aerobic endurance training decreases blood pressure through a reduction of vascular resistance, in which the sympathetic nervous system and the renin-angiotensin system appear to be involved, and favorably affects concomitant cardiovascular risk factors.

Static exercise

Blood pressure increases during acute static exercise and the increase is more pronounced than with dynamic exercise, particularly with heavy static exercise at an intensity of more than 40% to 50% of maximal voluntary contraction. In a recent meta-analysis of randomized controlled trials, "resistance" training at moderate intensity was found to decrease blood pressure by 3.5/3.2 mmHg [37]. The meta-analysis included nine studies designed to increase muscular strength and power or endurance, and all but one study involved dynamic, rather than purely static, exercise. In fact, few sports are characterized by purely static efforts. However, only three trials in the meta-analysis reported on patients who had hypertension.

Recommendations

General recommendations

Athletes with hypertension should be treated according to the general guidelines for the management of hypertension [1,14]. Appropriate nonpharmacologic measures should be considered in all patients (ie, moderate salt restriction, increase in fruit and vegetable intake, decrease in saturated and total fat intake, limitation of alcohol consumption to no more than 20 to 30 g ethanol/d for men and no more than 10 to 20 g ethanol/d for women, smoking cessation, and control of body weight). Antihypertensive drug therapy should be started promptly in patients at high or very high added risk for cardiovascular complications (see Table 2). In patients at low or moderate added risk, drug treatment is only initiated when hypertension persists after several weeks (moderate added risk) or months (low added risk) despite appropriate lifestyle changes. The goal of antihypertensive therapy is to reduce blood pressure to at least below 140/90 mm Hg, and to lower values if tolerated, in all hypertensive patients, and to below 130/80 mm Hg in diabetics and other high- or very high-risk conditions.

Current evidence indicates that patients who have white-coat hypertension do not have to be treated with antihypertensive drugs, unless they are at high or very high risk (see Table 2), but regular follow-up and nonpharmacologic measures are recommended [1,14]. Also, subjects with normal blood pressure at rest but exaggerated blood pressure response to exercise should be followed up more closely.

Choice of drugs

Several drug classes can be considered for the initiation of antihypertensive therapy: diuretics; beta-blockers; calcium channel blockers; angiotensin-converting enzyme inhibitors, and angiotensin II receptor blockers [1,14]. However, diuretics and beta-blockers are not recommended for first-line treatment in patients engaged in competitive or high-intensity endurance exercise [32]. Diuretics impair exercise performance and capacity in the first weeks of treatment through a reduction in plasma volume, but exercise tolerance appears to be restored during longer-term treatment; nevertheless, diuretics may cause electrolyte and fluid disturbances, which are not desirable in the endurance athlete. Beta-blockers reduce maximal aerobic power by 7% on average, as a result of the reduction in maximal heart rate, which is not fully compensated for by increases in maximal stroke volume, peripheral oxygen extraction, or both. Furthermore, the time that submaximal exercise can be sustained is reduced by about 20% by cardioselective beta-blockers and by about 40% by nonselective beta-blockers, most likely as a result of impaired lipolysis [32,38,39]. In addition, diuretics and beta-blockers are on the doping list for some sports in which weight loss or control of tremor are of paramount importance. Diuretics are also banned because they may be used to conceal the use of other doping agents, such as anabolic steroids, by diluting the urine samples. The hypertensive athlete who has to use a diuretic or beta-blocker for therapeutic purposes should follow the International Standard for Therapeutic Use Exceptions of the World Anti-Doping Agency.

Calcium channel blockers and blockers of the renin-angiotensin system are currently the drugs of choice for the hypertensive endurance athlete [32,40], and may be combined in case of insufficient blood pressure control. However, the combination of an angiotensin-converting enzyme inhibitor and an angiotensin II receptor blocker is currently not advocated for the treatment of hypertension because the benefit of the combination for blood pressure control has not been proved. If a third drug is required, a low-dose thiazide-like diuretic, possibly in combination with a potassium-sparing agent, is recommended. Unequivocal evidence that antihypertensive agents would impair performance in "resistance" sports does not exist.

Recommendations for leisure-time and competitive sports participation

Recommendations to athletes with hypertension for participation in intense leisure-time and competitive sports are based on the results of the evaluation and on the risk stratification (see Table 2), with the understanding that the general recommendations for the management of hypertension as described earlier are observed, and provided that the clinical condition is stable. Table 4 summarizes recommendations with regard to competitive sports participation [28,29].

The same recommendations may apply to patients who aim to engage in hard or very hard leisure-time sports activities to enhance performance substantially. However, most recreational physical activities are performed at low-to-moderate intensity. Dynamic sports activities are preferred, but also, low-to-moderate resistance training may not be harmful and may even contribute to blood pressure control [37]. In cases of cardiovascular or renal complications, the recommendations are based on the associated clinical conditions. Finally, all patients should be

Table 4
Recommendation for intense leisure-time physical activity and competitive sports participation in athletes who have systemic hypertension (and other risk factors) according to the cardiovascular risk profile

Risk category	Evaluation	Criteria for eligibility	Recommendations	Follow-up
Low added risk	History, PE, ECG, ET, Echo	Well-controlled BP	All sports	Yearly
Moderate added risk	History, PE, ECG, ET, Echo	Well-controlled BP and risk factors	All sports, with exclusion of high-static, high-dynamic sports (III C)	Yearly
High added risk	History, PE, ECG, ET, Echo	Well-controlled BP and risk factors	All sports, with exclusion of high-static sports (III A–C)	Yearly
Very high added risk	History, PE, ECG, ET, Echo	Well-controlled BP and risk factors; no associated clinical conditions	Only low- to moderate-dynamic, low-static sports (I A–B)	6 months

Abbreviations: BP, blood pressure; ECG, 12-lead electrocardiography; Echo, echocardiography at rest; ET, exercise testing; PE, physical examination, including repeated blood pressure measurements according to guidelines.

followed up at regular intervals, depending on the severity of hypertension and the category of risk (see Table 4). In addition, all exercising patients should be advised on exercise-related warning symptoms, such as chest pain or discomfort, abnormal dyspnea, and dizziness or malaise, which would necessitate consulting a qualified physician.

Summary

Hypertension is rare in the young, but its prevalence increases with aging. The overall risk of the hypertensive patient depends not only on blood pressure but also on the presence of other cardiovascular risk factors, target organ damage, and associated clinical conditions. The recommendations for preparticipation screening, sports participation, and follow-up depend on the cardiovascular risk profile of the individual athlete. When antihypertensive treatment is required, calcium channel blockers and blockers of the renin-angiotensin system are currently the drugs of choice.

Acknowledgments

The authors gratefully acknowledge the secretarial assistance of N. Ausseloos.

References

[1] Guidelines Committee. 2003 European Society of Hypertension–European Society of Cardiology guidelines for the management of arterial hypertension. J Hypertens 2003;21:1011–53.

[2] McKearney PM, Whelton M, Reynolds K, et al. Global burden of hypertension: analysis of worldwide data. Lancet 2005;365:217–23.

[3] Verdecchia P. Prognostic value of ambulatory blood pressure: current evidence and clinical implications. Hypertension 2000;35:844–51.

[4] Celis H, Fagard RH. White-coat hypertension: a clinical review. Eur J Intern Med 2004;15:348–57.

[5] Kouidi E, Fahadidou A, Tassoulas E, et al. White-coat hypertension detected during screening of male adolescent athletes. Am J Hypertens 1999;12:223–6.

[6] Björklund K, Lind L, Zethelius B, et al. Isolated ambulatory hypertension predicts cardiovascular morbidity in elderly men. Circulation 2003;107:1297–302.

[7] Prospective Studies Collaboration. Age-specific relevance of usual blood pressure to vascular mortality: a meta-analysis of individual data for one million

adults in 61 prospective studies. Lancet 2002;360:1903–13.

[8] Fagard RH, Celis H. Prognostic significance of various characteristics of out-of-the-office blood pressure. J Hypertens 2004;22:1663–6.

[9] Ohkubo T, Kikuya M, Metoki H, et al. Prognosis of masked hypertension and white-coat hypertension detected by 24-h ambulatory blood pressure monitoring. J Am Coll Cardiol 2005;46:508–15.

[10] Fagard RH, Van Den Broeke C, Decort P. Prognostic significance of blood pressure measured in the office, at home and during ambulatory monitoring in older patients in general practice. J Hum Hypertens 2005;19:801–7.

[11] Blood Pressure Lowering Treatment Trialists' Collaboration. Effects of different blood pressure-lowering regimens on major cardiovascular events: results of prospectively designed overviews of randomized trials. Lancet 2003;362:1527–35.

[12] EUROASPIRE II Study Group. Lifestyle and risk factor management and use of drug therapies in coronary patients from 15 countries. Principal results from EUROASPIRE II Euro Heart Survey Programme. Eur Heart J 2001;22:554–72.

[13] Fagard RH, Van den Enden M, Leeman M, et al. Survey on treatment of hypertension and implementation of WHO/ISH risk stratification in primary care in Belgium. J Hypertens 2002;20:1297–302.

[14] The Task Force of the Management of Arterial Hypertension of the European Society of Hypertension (ESH) and of the European Society of Cardiology (ESC). 2007 Guidelines for the Management of Arterial Hypertension. Journal of Hypertension 2007;25:1105–87.

[15] O'Brien, Asmar R, Beilin L, et al. European Society of Hypertension recommendations for conventional, ambulatory and home blood pressure measurement. J Hypertens 2003;21:821–48.

[16] Deligiannis A, Björnstad H, Carré F, et al. ESC Study Group of Sports Cardiology position paper on adverse cardiovascular effects of doping in athletes. Eur J Cardiovasc Prev Rehabil 2006;13:687–94.

[17] De Backer G, Ambrosioni E, Borck-Johnsen K, et al. European guidelines on cardiovascular disease prevention in clinical practice. Eur Heart J 2003;24:1601–10.

[18] Lewis JF, Spirito P, Pelliccia A, et al. Usefulness of Doppler echocardiographic assessment of diastolic filling in distinguishing 'athlete's heart' from hypertrophic cardiomyopathy. Br Heart J 1992;68:296–300.

[19] Pluim BM, Zwindermans AH, van der Laarse A, et al. The athlete's heart. A meta-analysis of cardiac structure and function. Circulation 1999;100:336–44.

[20] Fagard RH. The athlete's heart. Heart 2003;89:1455–61.

[21] Maron BJ, Pelliccia A. The heart of trained athletes. Cardiac remodeling and the risks of sports, including sudden death. Circulation 2006;114:1633–44.

[22] Devereux RB, Bella J, Boman K, et al. Echocardiographic left ventricular geometry in hypertensive patients with electrocardiographic left ventricular hypertrophy. The LIFE study. Blood Press 2001; 10:74–82.

[23] Maron BJ, Roberts WC, McAllister HA, et al. Sudden death in young athletes. Circulation 1980;62:218–29.

[24] Basso C, Corrado D, Thiene G. Cardiovascular causes of sudden death in young individuals including athletes. Cardiol Rev 1999;7:127–35.

[25] Corrado D, Pelliccia A, Björnstadt HH, et al. Cardiovascular pre-participation screening of young competitive athletes for prevention of sudden death: proposal for a common European protocol. Eur Heart J 2005;26:516–24.

[26] Virmani R, Burke AP, Farb A, et al. Causes of sudden death in young and middle-aged competitive athletes. Cardiol Clin 1997;15:439–72.

[27] McLenachan JM, Henderson E, Morris KI, et al. Ventricular arrhythmias in patients with hypertensive left ventricular hypertrophy. N Engl J Med 1987;317:787–92.

[28] Pelliccia A, Fagard R, Björnstadt HH, et al. Recommendations for competitive sports participation in athletes with cardiovascular disease. A consensus document from the Study Group of Sports Cardiology of the Working Group of Cardiac Rehabilitation and Exercise Physiology, and the Working Group of Myocardial and Pericardial Diseases of the European Society of Cardiology. Eur Heart J 2005;26:1422–45.

[29] Fagard RH, Björnstad HH, Borjesson M, et al. ESC Study Group on Sports Cardiology recommendations for participation in leisure-time physical activities and competitive sports for patients with hypertension. Eur J Cardiovasc Prev Rehabil 2005;12:326–31.

[30] Pescatello LS, Franklin B, Fagard R, et al. American College of Sports Medicine Position Stand: exercise and hypertension. Med Sci Sports Exerc 2004;36: 533–53.

[31] Fagard RH, Pardaens K, Staessen JA, et al. Should exercise blood pressure be measured in clinical practice? J Hypertens 1998;16:1215–7.

[32] Fagard R, Amery A. Physical exercise in hypertension. In: Laragh J, Brenner B, editors. Hypertension: pathophysiology, diagnosis and management. 2nd edition. New York: Raven Press; 1995. p. 2669–81.

[33] Fagard RH, Cornelissen V. Physical activity, exercise, fitness and blood pressure. In: Battegay EJ, Lip GYH, Bakris GL, editors. Handbook of hypertension: principles and practice. Boca Raton: Taylor & Francis; 2005. p. 195–206.

[34] Fagard RH. Exercise characteristics and the blood pressure response to dynamic physical training. Med Sci Sports Exerc 2001;33(Suppl):S484–92.

[35] Whelton SP, Chin A, Xin X, et al. Effects of aerobic exercise on blood pressure: a meta-analysis of randomised, controlled trials. Ann Intern Med 2002;136: 493–503.

[36] Cornelissen VA, Fagard RH. Effects of endurance training on blood pressure, blood pressure regulating mechanisms and cardiovascular risk factors. Hypertension 2005;46:667–75.

[37] Cornelissen VA, Fagard RH. Effect of resistance training on resting blood pressure: a meta-analysis of randomized controlled trials. J Hypertens 2005; 23:251–9.

[38] Van Baak MA. Hypertension, beta-adrenergic blocking agents and exercise. Int J Sports Med 1994;15:112–5.

[39] Vanhees L, Defoor JGM, Schepers D, et al. Effects of bisoprolol and atenolol on endurance exercise capacity in healthy men. J Hypertens 2000;18: 35–43.

[40] Vanhees L, Fagard R, Lijnen P, et al. Effect of antihypertensive medication on endurance exercise capacity in hypertensive sportsmen. J Hypertens 1991;9:1063–8.

ELSEVIER
SAUNDERS

Cardiol Clin 25 (2007) 449–455

CARDIOLOGY
CLINICS

How to Manage Athletes with Ventricular Arrhythmias

Alessandro Biffi, MD

Institute of Sports Medicine and Science, Italian Olympic Committee, Largo P. Gabrielli, 1, 00197, Rome, Italy

Young competitive athletes are perceived by the general population to be the healthiest members of the society. The possibility that highly trained athletes may have a potentially serious cardiac condition that can predispose to life-threatening tachyarrhythmias or sudden cardiac death seems paradoxical. However, high-risk ventricular tachyarrhythmias and sudden cardiac death, although uncommon, are extremely visible events, because of the high profile of elite and professional athletes [1,2]. In athletes under the age of 30 years, the incidence of sudden death is low and, in most cases, occurs in individuals with inherited heart disease [3,4]. In older athletes, sudden death is more common and is generally caused by arrhythmias in the context of coronary artery disease [5].

Indeed, regular exercise training is associated with morphologic and functional cardiac changes that may create ambiguity with cardiac pathologic conditions, and differentiating the benign, exercise-induced physiologic changes from true pathologic conditions with risk of sudden death is critical for developing appropriate screening strategies to reduce these adverse events [6–8].

Prevalence of premature ventricular depolarizations

Premature ventricular depolarizations (PVDs) can be quite common in the athletic population. The prevalence ranges from 6% to 70 % in most 24-hour Holter ECG studies in athletes, and up to 25% of complex forms in selected populations (Table 1) [9–13]. The difference in prevalence of

ventricular tachyarrhythmias are likely related to the different methods of athlete selection in various studies, and to influence of chance in the prevalence when only small groups of subjects are recruited. Such wide variations do not enable precise conclusions to be drawn on the actual prevalence of ventricular arrhythmias in apparently healthy athletes. However, the rarity of complex forms seems to be a consistent observation in various 24-hour ECG studies. Still, over the past years there have been an increasing number of articles reporting complex ventricular arrhythmias, and even cases of unexpected sudden cardiac death, probably of arrhythmic origin, in trained athletes [14–16].

Clinical significance of premature ventricular depolarizations

The question of life-threatening arrhythmias is especially relevant when the athlete is diagnosed to have an inherited genetic disorder (channelopathy) that may predispose to malignant ventricular arrhythmias [17–19]. For such reason, complex forms of ventricular arrhythmias in athletes continue to be an intriguing and prognostic dilemma for the cardiologists.

The following points summarize the most controversial clinical aspects:

1. The prevalence of ventricular arrhythmias in athletes without cardiovascular abnormalities is extremely variable, and the complex forms, such as idiopathic ventricular tachycardia (right or left ventricular outflow tract VT), appear to be very uncommon.
2. It is often difficult to identify a pathological cardiac substrate as possible cause of the

E-mail address: a.biffi@libero.it

0733-8651/07/$ - see front matter © 2007 Elsevier Inc. All rights reserved.
doi:10.1016/j.ccl.2007.07.007

Table 1

Prevalence of premature ventricular depolarizations on 24-hour Holter ECG monitoring in healthy athletes

Authors	Ref.	Year	Population (n =)	PVDs (%)	Complex PVDs (%)
H.Paparo	[11]	1981	32	6.2	0
Viitasalo	[9]	1982	35	28	5.7
Talan	[10]	1982	20	70	20
Palatini	[12]	1985	20	70	25
Italian Society of Sports Cardiology	[13]	1987	407	32	4.4

arrhythmia, even with the help of a growing number of noninvasive and invasive diagnostic testing.

3. It is not always easy (and ethically controversial) to suggests invasive tests, such as electrophysiologic study, endomyocardial biopsy, or coronary and ventricle angiography to an asymptomatic athlete only for assessing the origin and clinical significance of frequent PVDs

4. Physical exercise and training may represent a trigger for ominous ventricular tachyarrhythmias in athletes with underlying cardiovascular disease [20]

5. Long-term follow-up studies describing the clinical significance of frequent and complex ventricular arrhythmias in athletes are rare [21]

Before considering PVDs (or complex ventricular arrhythmias) as a benign expression of cardiac adaptation to exercise, physicians should search diligently for underlying structural heart diseases, particularly coronary artery disease (in adult individuals over 35 years old), right ventricular dysplasia, congenital coronary anomalies, hypertrophic or dilated cardiomyopathy, myocarditis, and catecholaminergic polymorphic ventricular tachycardia (in young individuals).

PVDs are reported to be associated with cardiovascular abnormalities in about 7% of athletes, but the likelihood of underlying cardiac disease is higher in those athletes with greater than 2,000 PVDs per 24 hour period than in those with less frequent PVDs (Fig. 1) [21]. Nevertheless, in the author's experience, over an 8-year follow-up period the risk of sudden cardiac death was exceedingly low (ie, 0.3%; annual mortality of 0.17%) [21].

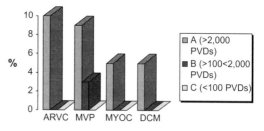

Fig. 1. Prevalence of structural cardiovascular abnormalities in elite athletes with ventricular arrhythmias. A = Athletes with more than 2,000 PVDs and more than 1 nonsustained ventricular tachycardia per 24 hour period; B = Athletes with more than 100 but fewer than 2,000 PVDs per 24 hour period; C = Athletes with fewer than 100 PVDs per 24 hour period. ARVC, arrhythmogenic right ventricular cardiomyopathy; MVP, mitral valve prolapse; MYOC, myocarditis; DCM, dilated cardiomyopathy; PVDs, premature ventricular depolarizations.

Assessment of premature ventricular depolarizations

Investigations include medical history, both personal history (palpitations, dyspnea or atypical chest pain, dizziness, unusual fatigue, syncope, and presyncope particularly if occurring during exercise) and familial history (premature sudden death in close relatives), physical examination, 12-lead ECG, ambulatory ECG monitoring, echocardiography, and exercise testing.

Frequent and complex PVDs on Holter, or an increase in the frequency of PVDs during physical exercise, as well as subjective palpitations or symptoms of hemodynamic impairment, should prompt a more extensive cardiovascular evaluation, including cardiac magnetic resonance (CMR), cardiac catheterization, or endomyocardial biopsy, when appropriate. In fact, presence of cardiovascular abnormalities, in particular of the right ventricle origin, have been recently demonstrated in association with ventricular arrhythmias and were identified by performing cardiac angiography, endomyocardial biopsy, or cine-CMR [22,23]. However, the difficulty to correctly identify the arrhythmic substrate is exemplified by the fact that a more careful morphologic evaluation of athletes with ventricular arrhythmias, in the absence of apparent heart disease at usual noninvasive investigations, showed the presence of focal thinning and fatty replacements of the outflow tract, or functional impairment of the right ventricle in athletes versus control subjects [22]. This impairment was reflected in a significantly lower right ventricular ejection fraction and outflow tract-shortening fraction. Such predilection of ventricular arrhythmias for the right ventricle in athletes is also documented by the morphology of the PVDs, like left bundle branch block, frequently associated with vertical axis. This morphology commonly occurs also in athletes without cardiovascular abnormalities (ie, 70% of cases in the author's experience) [21].

The differentiation between idiopathic and pathologic ventricular arrhythmias is even more relevant in athletes who show structural cardiac adaptations and electrophysiologic changes as part of the "athlete's heart"[24]. Some investigators suspect that endurance sports by itself may lead to right ventricular structural enlargement and possible electrical changes that might not have developed without the activity [22]. Long-lasting volume overload has been suggested as the mechanism contributing to the development of such right ventricular changes.

On the other hand, several studies, also including CMR, concluded that regular and extensive endurance training results in symmetric changes in left and right ventricular dimensions and volume, confirming the concept that the athlete's heart is a balanced, enlarged, and normally functioning heart [25]. Indeed, considering the large number of athletes with ventricular arrhythmias and their favorable clinical outcome, it seems unlikely such rare genetic diseases or minor right ventricular abnormalities could be responsible for the large proportion of ventricular arrhythmias observed in the athletes. Furthermore, recent advances in laboratory DNA analysis have demonstrated a genetic basis for some arrhythmogenic syndromes unassociated with left ventricular hypertrophy (ie, long QT syndrome, Brugada syndrome, and catecholaminergic polymorphic ventricular tachycardia). These arrhythmias may be life threatening in young adults in association with even recreational sports activities. It is not possible, therefore, to definitively exclude the possibility that such uncommon genetic disorders represent a small proportion of apparently healthy athletes presenting with ventricular tachyarrhythmias.

Electrophysiologic (EP) study with programmed ventricular stimulation is generally ineffective in athletes without cardiovascular abnormalities. In the 13 athletes with frequent and complex ventricular arrhythmias of the author's previous investigation, either no arrhythmia or

only nonsustained responses were induced during the EP test [21]. The predictive accuracy of this technique for future arrhythmic events is very low in the apparently healthy athletic population, as compared with patients with coronary artery disease.

However, EP study may be useful to assess the arrhythmia's mechanism in the prospective of a catheter ablation [26]: there is evidence that re-entry tachyarrhythmias confer a more ominous prognosis when they occur in structurally abnormal myocardium, and have the potential for development of life-threatening arrhythmias. On the other hand, automatic and unifocal arrhythmias may be idiopathic and are usually clinically benign [15]. Spontaneous ventricular tachycardia with rates below 100 to 150 beats per minute are generally focal and have a good prognosis in the absence of underlying heart disease. Idiopathic ventricular arrhythmias (as from right ventricular outflow tract- origin or fascicular-VT) and some other automatic VTs are amenable to radiofrequency catheter ablation, with a reasonable success rate. The procedures, however, carry a small risk of adverse effects (perforation, thrombo-embolism among others), which should be clearly discussed in advance with the athlete.

Signal-averaged electrocardiogram for detecting the presence of ventricular late potentials shows a low predictive value for future arrhythmic events in trained athletes, but a higher prevalence of late potentials in athletes with ventricular tachyarrhythmias have been reported, as compared with sedentary controls [27].

Work-up should also include a search for agents that might enhance ventricular irritability, such as use of excessive amounts of alcohol, illicit drugs, or stimulants, particularly ephedrine and caffeine. In female athletes, fluctuating levels of estrogen hormones that occur during the menstrual cycle, during pregnancy or menopause, or with birth control pills, may cause PVDs to appear.

The impact of sports on ventricular arrhythmias

A crucial point is the role played by physical exercise and training in the genesis of ventricular arrhythmias and, therefore, whether exercise can enhance the risk of arrhythmic cardiac arrest in athletes. Corrado and colleagues [20] showed that the risk for sudden death in young competitive athletes with cardiovascular disease (mostly of arrhythmic origin) was 2.5-fold greater than in nonathletes. These data suggest that sports activity itself may act as a trigger for life-threatening ventricular tachyarrhythmias in susceptible individuals who have underlying, even silent cardiovascular disease.

These findings are in agreement with results of the author's previous study on physical deconditioning, in which it was observed that none of the 50 athletes with frequent and complex ventricular arrhythmias (with or without cardiovascular abnormalities) disqualified from training and competition, experienced clinical events or cardiac arrest in the follow-up and, on the contrary, showed a marked reduction or even disappearance of the PVDs (Fig. 2) [28]. Therefore, the reduction or disappearance of ventricular arrhythmias is a potential mechanism by which disqualification from competitive sports may reduce the risk for sudden cardiac death [6–8].

These data support the restriction from competitive sport and intense exercise training in athletes with frequent and complex ventricular arrhythmias and structural heart disease, as stated by current recommendations for managing athletes with arrhythmias [26,29–31]. Therefore, polymorphic and malignant ventricular tachycardia triggered by intensive athletic conditioning should raise suspicion and greater scrutiny for an underlying inherited electrophysiologic disorder (such as channelopathies), or an underlying structural disease (such as arrhythmogenic right ventricular dysplasia or hypertrophic cardiomyopathy).

Athletes with ventricular arrhythmias and no cardiovascular abnormalities

The most difficult group, with regard to clinical management, consists of athletes with frequent and complex ventricular arrhythmias in the absence of structural heart disease. The author's

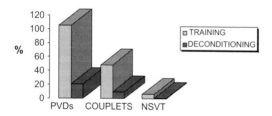

Fig. 2. Reduction of ventricular tachyarrhythmias after deconditioning. NSVT, nonsustained ventricular tachycardia.

longitudinal follow-up data are persuasive in supporting the view that ventricular tachyarrhythmias appear benign and do not require alteration in athletic lifestyle, in particular in athletes with less than 2,000 PVDs per 24 hour period and no episode of nonsustained ventricular tachycardia [21]. It would appear that such arrhythmias in the absence of underlying structural heart disease, even in athletes subjected to the unique environmental conditions and stress of intense sports training and competition, do not convey an ominous prognosis. If any, ventricular arrhythmias in some athletes without apparent cardiovascular abnormalities, would appear to represent another expression of the autonomic nervous system changes associated with the "athlete's heart" (such as bradycardia or atrio-ventricular conduction disturbances).

Nevertheless, some investigators suspect that it is not always possible to distinguish marked myocardial changes, expression of a physiologic adaptation to physical training, from those associated with an early stage of cardiomyopathy [16,22]. Such considerations appear of particular relevance in the presence of frequent and complex ventricular tachyarrhythmias. In particular, it is not known whether myocardial hypertrophy induced by exercise training may also induce cellular electrical changes that represent a possible trigger for ventricular arrhythmias in certain athletes, potentially increasing their cardiovascular risk. Although this relationship cannot be excluded in any single athlete, a recent investigation shows that left ventricular (LV) remodeling (ie, increase in cavity dimension, wall thickness, and mass) is not related to the presence and frequency of ventricular arrhythmias in elite athletes free of cardiovascular abnormalities [32]. Paradoxically, trained athletes with the smallest amount of LV remodeling demonstrate a propensity to more frequent ventricular arrhythmias. This observation makes evident that training-induced myocardial hypertrophy does not convey, per se, an increased risk for ventricular arrhythmogenesis. These data were also supported by results of the previous study performed in athletes with ventricular tachyarrhythmias who underwent a period of deconditioning, which showed a similar decrease in cardiac dimensions in athletes with and without reversible ventricular arrhythmias [28].

These results are in contrast with the hypothesis that cellular electrophysiologic changes induced by cardiac hypertrophy were sufficient to account for many of the abnormalities in the athlete's ECG, including high-grade ventricular ectopy [33]. According to this hypothesis, sudden death in trained athletes (in the absence of demonstrable heart disease) may be a direct consequence of cardiac hypertrophy itself and abnormal repolarization behavior induced by hypertrophy. However, and most relevant, the tissue and cellular changes characteristic of pathologic hypertrophy are not the same of the exercise-induced hypertrophy. Recent findings in animal models with myocardial hypertrophy have provided the molecular basis for a concept, which favors the existence of either compensatory or maladaptive forms of hypertrophy [34]. To date, a few experimental studies have been published describing changes in specific current systems in myocytes isolated from the hearts of animals subjected to exercise training. These studies showed no changes in Calcium (Ca^2+) current characteristics in trained animals [35]. Further studies are required to assess the changes in cellular electrophysiology, in particular to define the detailed cellular mechanisms for arrhythmias at a different stage of hypertrophy. Therefore, other causes of arrhythmias, such as autonomic nervous system or genetic changes, should be examined to explain the reversibility of ventricular arrhythmias after deconditioning.

Recommendations for sports participation

The recommendations regarding sports participation of athletes with ventricular tachyarrhythmias have been recently published [26,29–31]. In athletes with these rhythm disturbances and evidence of cardiovascular abnormalities, participation in sports is generally dependent on the underlying cardiac condition. Participation in sports is generally allowed and unrestricted in athletes without cardiac disease or primary arrhythmogenic conditions, without family history of sudden death and symptoms, and when arrhythmias are not related to exercise. Yearly follow-up and revaluation is generally suggested for such athletes [26,30]. In the majority of athletes with frequent PVDs, deconditioning for 3 to 6 months may result in a substantial decrease of arrhythmias, thereby confirming the favorable prognosis.

Treatment

Athletes without cardiovascular abnormalities

Usually, only ventricular tachyarrhythmias associated with normal hearts are currently curable. However, frequent and complex ventricular ectopy, in the absence of underlying structural heart disease, is generally of benign nature and does not need drug therapy. If arrhythmic symptoms (ie, palpitations) cannot be controlled by deconditioning, then drug therapy in form of beta-blockade or calcium channel blockade may be considered. However, the use of beta-blockade is not permitted in the majority of sports (those drugs are included in the World Anti-Doping Agency list of doping substances). Alternatives to beta-blockade include calcium channel blockade in the form of diltiazem or verapamil. In the case of isolated right ventricular outflow tachycardia, easily inducible by electrophysiologic testing, especially with the use of isoproterenol, radiofrequency ablation can be indicated [36]. Return to competitive sport is usually allowed after at least one month from successful ablation, provided that arrhythmia is not more inducible after the ablation procedure.

Athletes with cardiovascular abnormalities

In patients with underlying structural heart disease, the cure is addressed to the primary cardiac condition. In fact, radiofrequency ablation of ventricular arrhythmias in the presence of heart disease does not guarantee a protection against sudden cardiac death. In patients with heart disease (such as coronary artery disease, hypertrophic cardiomyopathy, arrhythmogenic right ventricular dysplasia, channelopathies, and others) several strategies have been developed and include surgery, beta-blockers, antiarrhythmic agents, permanent pacemakers, radiofrequency ablation, and implantable cardioverter defibrillators (ICDs). Restriction from competitive sports is recommended for athletes with heart disease and syncope, in particular during exercise, or resuscitated sudden cardiac death. In the individual with ventricular arrhythmias and idiopathic cardiomyopathy, beta-blockers and angiotensin-converting enzyme inhibitors lower the risk of all cause mortality and sudden death and should be prescribed in all patients. In patients with coronary artery disease and ventricular arrhythmias, ICDs give the best protection against sudden death [37].

Summary

In conclusion, premature ventricular depolarizations in trained athletes are generally of benign nature and, if there is no evidence of underlying structural heart disease, they are generally not treated with drug therapy and should not be viewed as an obstacle for participation in athletic training and competition.

References

[1] Maron BJ, Shirani J, Poliac LC, et al. Sudden death in young competitive athletes. Clinical, demographics, and pathological profiles. JAMA 1996;276: 199–204.

[2] Van Camp SP, Bloor CM, Mueller FO, et al. Non-traumatic sports death in high school and college athletes. Med Sci Sports Exerc 1995;27:641–7.

[3] Maron BJ. Sudden death in young athletes. N Engl J Med 2003;349:1308–20.

[4] Corrado D, Basso C, Schiavon M, et al. Screening for hypertrophic cardiomyopathy in young athletes. N Engl J Med 1998;339:364–9.

[5] Waller BF, Roberts WC. Sudden death while running in conditioned runners aged 40 years or over. Am J Cardiol 1980;45:1292–7.

[6] Corrado D, Pelliccia A, Bjørnstad HH, et al. Cardiovascular pre-participation screening of young competitive athletes for prevention of sudden death: proposal for a common European protocol. Eur Heart J 2005;26:516–24.

[7] Pelliccia A, Di Paolo FM, Corrado D, et al. Evidence for efficacy of the Italian national pre-participation screening program for identification of hypertrophic cardiomyopathy in competitive athletes. Eur Heart J 2006;27:2196–200.

[8] Corrado D, Basso C, Pavei A, et al. Trends in sudden cardiovascular death in young competitive athletes after implementation of a pre-participation screening program. JAMA 2006;296:1593–601.

[9] Viitaasalo MT, Kala R, Eisalo A. Ambulatory electrocardiographic recording in endurance athletes. Br Heart J 1982;47:213–20.

[10] Talan DA, Bauernfeind RA, Ashley WW, et al. Twenty-four hour continuous ECG recordings in long-distance runners. Chest 1982;82:19–24.

[11] Hanne Paparo N, Kellermann JJ. Long-term Holter ECG monitoring in athletes. Med Sci Sports Exerc 1981;13:294–8.

[12] Palatini P, Maraglino G, Sperti G, et al. Prevalence and possible mechanisms of ventricular arrhythmias in athletes. Am Heart J 1985;110:560–7.

[13] Italian Society of Sports Cardiology. Standards of dynamic electrocardiography (Holter) in top-ranking athletes of different sports. In: Lubich T, Venerando A, Zeppilli P, editors. Sports Cardiology. 2nd edition. Bologna, Italy: Aulo Gaggi; 1989. p. 355–61.

[14] Durakovic Z, Misigoj-Durakovic M, Vuori I, et al. Sudden cardiac death due to physical exercise in male competitive athletes. A report of six cases. J Sports Med Phys Fitness 2005;45:532–6.

[15] Heidbuchel H, Hoogsteen J, Fagard R, et al. High prevalence of right ventricular involvement in endurance athletes with ventricular arrhythmias. Role of an electrophysiologic study in risk stratification. Eur Heart J 2003;24:1473–80.

[16] Furlanello F, Bertoldi A, Dallago M, et al. Cardiac arrest and sudden death in competitive athletes with arrhythmogenic right ventricular dysplasia. Pacing Clin Electrophysiol 1998;21:331–4.

[17] Moss AJ. Long QT syndrome. JAMA 2003;289: 2041–4.

[18] Antzelevitch C, Brugada P, Borggrefe M, et al. Brugada syndrome: report of the second consensus conference. Heart Rhythm 2005;2:1648–54.

[19] D'Amati G, Bagattin A, Bauce B, et al. Juvenile sudden death in a family with polymorphic ventricular arrhythmias caused by a novel RyR2 gene mutation: evidence of specific morphological substrates. Hum Pathol 2005;36:761–7.

[20] Corrado D, Basso C, Rizzoli G, et al. Does sports activity enhance the risk of sudden death in adolescents and young adults? J Am Coll Cardiol 2003;42: 1959–63.

[21] Biffi A, Pelliccia A, Verdile L, et al. Long-term clinical significance of frequent and complex ventricular tachyarrhythmias in trained athletes. J Am Coll Cardiol 2002;40:446–52.

[22] Ector J, Ganame J, Van der Merwe N, et al. Reduced right ventricular ejection fraction in endurance athletes presenting with ventricular arrhythmias: a quantitative angiographic assessment. Eur Heart J 2007;28:345–53.

[23] Globits S, Kreiner G, Frank H, et al. Significance of morphological abnormalities detected by MRI in patients undergoing successful ablation of right ventricular outflow tachycardia. Circulation 1997;96: 2633–40.

[24] Pelliccia A, Maron BJ, Culasso F, et al. Clinical significance of abnormal electrocardiographic patterns in trained athletes. Circulation 2000;102:278–84.

[25] Scharhag J, Schneider G, Urhausen A, et al. Athlete's heart: right and left ventricular mass and function in male endurance athletes and untrained individuals determined by magnetic resonance imaging. J Am Coll Cardiol 2002;40:1856–63.

[26] Heidbuchel H, Corrado D, Biffi A, et al. Recommendations for participation in leisure-time physical activity and competitive sports of patients with arrhythmias and potentially arrhythmogenic conditions. Part II: ventricular arrhythmias, channelopathies and implantable defibrillators. Eur J Cardiovasc Prev Rehabil 2006;13:876–86.

[27] Biffi A, Ansalone G, Verdile L, et al. Ventricular arrhythmias and athlete's heart: role of signal-averaged electrocardiography. Eur Heart J 1996;17:557–63.

[28] Biffi A, Maron BJ, Verdile L, et al. Impact of physical deconditioning on ventricular tachyarrhythmias in trained athletes. J Am Coll Cardiol 2004;44: 1053–8.

[29] Maron BJ, Zipes DP. 36th Bethesda Conference: Introduction: eligibility recommendations for competitive athletes with cardiovascular abnormalities-general considerations. J Am Coll Cardiol 2005;45:1318–21.

[30] Pelliccia A, Fagard R, Bjørnstad HH, et al. Recommendations for competitive sports participation in athletes with cardiovascular disease. Eur Heart J 2005;26:1422–45.

[31] Italian cardiological guidelines for competitive sports eligibility (COCIS). J Sports Cardiol 2005;2:24–43.

[32] Biffi A, Maron BJ, Porcacchia P, et al. The paradox of ventricular tachyarrhythmias and left ventricular mass in athlete's heart [abstract]. Circulation 2005; 112:II-396.

[33] Hart G. Exercise-induced cardiac hypertrophy: a substrate for sudden death in athletes? Exp Physiol 2003;88(5):639–44.

[34] Lips DJ, deWindt LJ, Van Kraaij DJ, et al. Molecular determinants of myocardial hypertrophy and failure: alternative pathways for beneficial and maladaptive hypertrophy. Eur Heart J 2003;24: 883–96.

[35] Mokelke EA, Palmer BM, Cheung JY, et al. Endurance training does not affect intrinsic calcium current characteristics in rat myocardium. Am J Physiol 1997;273:H1193–7.

[36] Stevenson WG. Catheter ablation of monomorphic ventricular tachycardia. Curr Opin Cardiol 2005; 20:42–7.

[37] AVID Investigators. A comparison of antiarrhythmic-drug therapy with implantable defibrillators in patients resuscitated from near-fatal ventricular arrhythmias. N Engl J Med 1997; 337:1576–83.

ELSEVIER
SAUNDERS

Cardiol Clin 25 (2007) 457–466

CARDIOLOGY
CLINICS

How to Manage Athletes with Syncope

Mark S. Link, MD*, N.A. Mark Estes III, MD

*The New England Cardiac Arrhythmia Center, Division of Cardiology, Tufts-New England Medical Center,
Box #197, 750 Washington Street, Boston, MA 02111, USA*

Syncope is defined as transient loss of consciousness accompanied by loss of postural tone. Episodes are typically brief, but can last up to several minutes in some individuals. In these prolonged episodes of syncope, cardiopulmonary resuscitation could be performed by an astute observer. The individual then awakens, not secondary to cardiopulmonary resuscitation but to the spontaneous resumption of blood pressure [1,2]. Presyncope is described as a feeling of lightheadedness that nearly causes collapse, while dizziness is a less well defined symptom that can be characterized by any sort of abnormal sensation in the head or body.

Syncope in the setting of exercise may be secondary to underlying cardiac disease and thus predictive of sudden cardiac death (SCD). In a retrospective study of all sudden, nontraumatic deaths occurring over a period of 12 years in young Israeli soldiers (n = 44, age range 17–22 years), it was found that 23% had experienced at least one episode of syncope before death. The syncopal events occurred between 1 hour and 4 years before death. In 16%, the syncopal episode had occurred during exercise [3]. Maron and colleagues [4] reported an incidence of syncope or presyncope of 17% in a cohort of 29 young athletes who subsequently died suddenly.

In general, a competitive athlete is defined as one who participates in a sport requiring systematic training and regular competition against others, either on an individual basis or in an organized team [5,6]. It has been noted that an important facet of this group of individuals is the low likelihood of termination of exercise in the face of warning symptoms (such as presyncope or syncope), either because of the pressure of organized athletic competition, or because of an inability to consider the relevance of these symptoms.

Incidence

In the general population, syncope is seen in up to 40% over a lifetime. The authors have had little information on the incidence in the athlete until recently, when data from the Italian screening programs have become available. In this recent series, Colivicchi and colleagues reported on 7568 athletes screened for athletic participation [7]. In these, 474 (6.2%) reported a syncopal spell in the preceding 5 years. Syncope was unrelated to exercise in 87.7%, postexertional in 12.0%, and exertional in 1.3%. In subsequent follow-up, those with a prior history of syncope had a recurrence of 20 per 1000 subject-years, while those without a prior history of syncope had an occurrence of 2.2 per 1000 subject-years.

Risks of exercise

Although the long-term benefit of exercise has been shown to decrease the mortality of a number of diseases, this beneficial effect does not come without some acute risk. A number of investigators have shown that there is an increased risk of sudden death in athletes with underlying cardiovascular disease, including the young [8–11]. During exercise, mechanisms for the increased risk of sudden death include plaque rupture, caused by shear stress, and subsequent coronary thrombosis, increased arrhythmias caused by the increased work load of the heart and circulating catecholamines, and rupture of the great vessels [12,13].

---

* Corresponding author.
E-mail address: mlink@tufts-nemc.org (M.S. Link).

doi:10.1016/j.ccl.2007.07.005

Workup of the athlete with syncope

The athlete with syncope presents a unique challenge to the physician. Syncope in young individuals is usually benign; however, syncope can be a warning of impending SCD, especially in those with diagnosed or undiagnosed heart disease [14–17]. The etiology of syncope in these young healthy individuals ranges from benign neurocardiogenic syncope to nonsustained life-threatening arrhythmias. In these individuals, in whom most will have benign causes of syncope, it is critically important to identify those who may be at risk of a life-threatening disorder.

Presence of structural heart disease

As in the nonathlete, patients with no organic heart disease are at a low risk of sudden death. By contrast, the presence of structural heart disease is associated with an increased risk of sudden death. Thus, in the athlete with syncope, an echocardiogram is necessary in all but the most classic neurocardiogenic syndromes. In most North American series on sudden death in the young athlete, hypertrophic cardiomyopathy and anomalous coronary arteries are the most common underlying heart disease [16]. However, the experience in Italy is that arrhythmogenic right ventricular dysplasia (ARVD) is the most common underlying organic heart disease [18,19]. In general, it appears that those young patients with hypertrophic cardiomyopathy, ARVD, and anomalous origin of the coronary arteries are at the highest risk of life-threatening arrhythmias. Ventricular arrhythmias in the setting of congenital heart disease, such as Ebstein's anomaly, tetralogy of Fallot, and other stenotic or regurgitant valvular heart disease also indicates a higher risk of life-threatening arrhythmic events in the athlete [20]. Idiopathic dilated cardiomyopathy and acute myocarditis are also rare causes of sudden death. Understanding of commotio cordis has increased in the recent years, and it is presently the second leading cause of sudden death in athletes [16,21,22]. As the athlete ages, coronary artery disease becomes more common and accounts for a higher prevalence of heart disease. In the athlete over 30 years old, coronary artery disease is the underlying disease in up to 80% of patients.

History

The history in the evaluation of the athlete with symptoms of syncope or presyncope is paramount in the diagnosis (Table 1) [2,23–25].

Table 1
Clinical characteristics helpful in differentiating arrhythmic from nonarrhythmic syncope

	Neurocardiogenic or nonarrhythmic	Arrhythmic
Prodrome	Lightheadedness, warmth, nausea	None or brief lightheadedness
Number of episodes	Multiple	Few or one
Situational factors	Fear, fright, upright posture	Exertional, unrelated to posture
Post syncopal symptoms	Frequently fatigue	Usually none
Injury	Unusual	Common
Underlying heart disease	Unusual	Common

Data from Link MS, Wang PJ, Estes NA III. Ventricular arrhythmias in the athlete. Curr Opin Cardiol 2001;16:33.

Syncope or presyncope that occur during exertion are more likely to be life-threatening than those that occur at rest [18,20,26]. The Reggie Lewis death focused interest on exercise-induced neurocardiogenic syncope and several series of potential cases were published [27–30]. However, based on careful reading of these series and new data from Colivicchi [7], what is called exercise-induced neurocardiogenic syncope is in fact syncope that occurs after exercise or during pauses in exertion (ie, time outs or shooting foul shots). Postexertional syncope (such as standing at a foul line or during a time out) is not likely to be life-threatening, but is likely to be caused by vasodilatation and corresponding hypotension [7,31,32]. In one of the few epidemiologic series of syncope in athletes, Colivicchi reported that of 7,568 athletes screened in the Italian screening program, 474 reported syncope in the prior 5 years. In those who had syncope unrelated to exertion (86.7%), the diagnosis was either vasovagal or situational. In those who had syncope in association with exertion, the syncope was postexertional in 12%; cardiac workup was normal and in follow-up no sudden death occurred. However in those with syncope during exertion (n = 6, or 1.3%) hypertrophic cardiomyopathy and right ventricular ventricular tachycardia were seen in one each, while the remaining four had neurally-mediated syncope [7].

Syncope without prodromal symptoms is more troubling than a gradual onset of syncope. Syncope that occurs only with upright posture is less likely to be arrhythmic than that occurring during sitting or lying down. Syncope with clear and reproducible triggers of stress, excitement, or fear is more likely to be neurocardiogenic than arrhythmic. Injury secondary to syncope is more often seen in arrhythmic disorders and rarely seen in neurocardiogenic syncope, in which individuals often "slump" to the floor and thus are able to break their fall with their arms. Frequent episodes of presyncope and lightheadedness are less likely to be arrhythmic in origin than occasional episodes of syncope. Note should also be made of a family medical history of sudden death, especially at an early age. In individuals with this family history, syncope is more concerning in that it may be a harbinger of an inherited life-threatening cardiac condition.

In an athlete with symptoms consistent with ventricular arrhythmias (sudden onset, injury associated with syncope, exertionally related symptoms) a full evaluation is usually necessary [32]. In an athlete with symptoms suggestive of less serious conditions, such as dehydration, postexertional, or neurally mediated syncope (premonitory symptoms, gradual onset of syncope, frequent symptoms, nonexertional symptoms, orthostatic symptoms) little or no further evaluation may be needed. Because many of the structural heart diseases associated with sudden death are genetic in origin, athletes with a family history of early SCD require a thorough workup.

Electrocardiogram and loop monitoring

It is well recognized that abnormal ECGs are common in athletes (Table 2) [33,34]. The spectrum of abnormalities includes sinus bradycardia, first- and second-degree heart block, early repolarization, left ventricular hypertrophy, and T-wave inversion [35–37]. However, certain ECG abnormalities are associated with heart disease and an increased risk of life-threatening arrhythmias. These abnormalities include the pseudo-infarct pattern seen in hypertrophic cardiomyopathy (septal Q-waves) and Wolff-Parkinson-White syndrome (inferior Q-waves) [4,33,38]. ARVD patients typically have precordial T-wave inversion. In addition, these patients occasionally possess right ventricular conduction delays with a characteristic late depolarization of the right ventricle, known as the epsilon wave, or even complete right bundle branch block [39,40]. Long QT syndrome patients are diagnosed almost solely by ECG criteria [41–43].

Table 2
Electrocardiographic abnormalities found in various disease states

Diagnosis of heart disease	ECG abnormalities
Arrhythmogenic right ventricular dysplasia	T-wave inversions anteriorly Epsilon wave RBBB (complete or incomplete) Rarely normal
Hypertrophic cardiomyopathy	Left ventricular hypertrophy Pseudoinfarct with Q-waves anteriorly Rarely normal
Idiopathic dilated cardiomyopathy	LBBB Prolonged QT Can be normal
Long QT syndrome	Prolonged QT Abnormal appearance of ST segment
Brugada syndrome	RBBB (complete or incomplete) ST elevation anteriorly Changes can vary with time
Anomalous coronary artery	Typically no abnormalities
Coronary artery disease	Typically no abnormalities Q-waves ST segment abnormalities
Wolff-Parkinson-White syndrome	Short PR interval Delta waves Pseudoinfarct patterns

Data from Link MS, Wang PJ, Estes NA III. Ventricular arrhythmias in the athlete. Curr Opin Cardiol 2001;16:35.

Long-term ECG monitoring with Holter monitors can be useful in those patients with frequent or reproducible symptoms. Athletes with intermittent symptoms are best evaluated with a continuous loop monitor. These monitors continuously record a 1- to 3-minute segment of a surface electrocardiogram, and with activation by a button on the loop monitor the tape is frozen and the previous few minutes of the event are recorded.

Tilt-table testing

While tilt-table testing may not specifically identify the cause of syncope, this modality may determine an exaggerated susceptibility to normal reflex events leading to syncope. However, controversy remains regarding the sensitivity and specificity of tilt-table testing, with particular unease surrounding its use in athletes. Estimates of the accuracy of tilt testing have ranged between 30% and 80% [44,45]. In persons with neurocardiogenic syncope, up to 80% may have an abnormal result [45]. Concern over the broader use of tilt testing in athletes with an undefined cause for their syncope has centered around the observation that orthostatic stress may cause a positive result in athletes with no clinical history of syncope [45]. These false positive results may conceal other, more serious causes of syncope. Thus, there are mixed recommendations regarding tilt-table testing, ranging from advocating avoidance of tilt-table testing in athletes, to warning that the diagnostic ability of tilt testing is limited, to endorsing the use of this modality if the diagnosis of neurocardiogenic syncope is likely [44,46]. Results of tilt-table testing should thus not be solely relied upon to make a diagnosis.

Electrophysiologic observations

As in nonathletic populations, selected individuals with syncope should undergo an electrophysiologic evaluation (Table 3) [1,47]. Selection criteria are not always agreed upon; however, in general, if there is concern about supraventricular or ventricular tachyarrhythmias, invasive electrophysiologic testing should be performed. The electrophysiologic evaluation is of limited value in the assessment of bradyarrhythmias because of the poor sensitivity of the test. Specificity in the athlete may also be poor because of the influence of the high vagal tone seen in athletes.

The sensitivity and specificity of the electrophysiologic evaluation for supraventricular tachyarrhythmias are high. Underlying substrate for atrioventricular (AV) nodal re-entrant tachycardia and AV re-entrant tachycardias (those seen in Wolff-Parkinson-White syndrome) are readily diagnosed. In addition, induction of arrhythmia is generally accomplished in AV nodal re-entrant tachycardia, AV re-entrant tachycardia, and atrial tachycardia. Isoproterenol may be needed to facilitate induction. In the setting of an accessory bypass tract, it is important to assess for sudden

Table 3
Value of programmed stimulation in patients with spontaneous sustained ventricular tachycardia

Condition	Sensitivity	Specificity
Normal heart	+	+++
HCM	+	+
CAD	++++	++++
Anomalous CAD	No utility	No utility
ARVD	+++	+++
LQTS	No utility	No utility
IDCM	+	+
Idiopathic LV VT	+++	+++
Idiopathic RV VT	+++	+++

+-poor utility; ++-fair utility; +++-good utility; ++++-excellent utility.

ARVD, arrhythmogenic right ventricular dysplasia; CAD, coronary artery disease; HCM, hypertrophic cardiomyopathy; IDCM, idiopathic cardiomyopathy; LQTS, long QT syndrome; LV, left ventricle; RV, right ventricle; VT, ventricular tachycardia.

Data from Link MS, Estes NAM. Ventricular arrhythmias. In: Estes NAM, Salem DN, Wang PJ, editors. Sudden Cardiac Death in the Athlete. Futura Publishing Co., Armonk, NY, 1998. p. 258.

death risk. If the conduction through the accessory pathway is very rapid, the risk of ventricular fibrillation may be high [48]. Ability to conduct at heart rates of 240 or greater are thought to put the patient at an increased risk of sudden death, and ablation is recommended for these individuals [49–51].

Ventricular stimulation is of use primarily in those with scar related ventricular tachycardia, such as those patients with prior myocardial infarctions and possibly ARVD. In patients with coronary artery disease, ventricular stimulation is of reasonably high sensitivity (90%–95%) [52,53] and specificity (95% for induced monomorphic ventricular tachycardia) [53]. However, the significance of induced nonsustained ventricular tachycardia and ventricular fibrillation is less well established [54]. In patients with arrhythmogenic right ventricular dysplasia, the sensitivity of ventricular stimulation was thought to be 70% to 80% [55]; however, more recent data has suggested that ventricular stimulation may not be as useful as previously thought [56].

Unfortunately, the sensitivity and specificity of ventricular stimulation is low in patients with hypertrophic cardiomyopathy, idiopathic dilated cardiomyopathy, long QT syndrome, and congenital heart disease [57], diseases which are the most common in young individuals dying suddenly.

Causes and treatment of the athlete with syncope

Neurally mediated syncope

Neurocardiogenic syncope is the most common cause of syncope in the young individual. This disorder is characterized by occurring during upright posture, frequent situational triggers, and premonitory symptoms of warmth, lightheadedness, palpitations, sweating, and pallor. Loss of consciousness occurs over 5 to 10 seconds, often causing "slumping," although some episodes may be quite abrupt. Patients typically regain consciousness rapidly, but feelings of fatigue continue. More recently, it has become appreciated that neurocardiogenic syncope is but one of several neurally mediated syncope disorders, the others of which are autonomic failure, postural orthostatic tachycardia syndrome, and cerebral vasoconstrictive syncope [46,58,59].

The approach to the treatment of neurocardiogenic syncope is multifaceted. Initially all individuals should be advised to stay well hydrated and to liberalize their use of salt, even ingesting salt tablets if they do not wish to increase the salt content of their diet. Tilt training is a technique that has been demonstrated in some studies to be efficacious in the treatment of neurocardiogenic syncope [60]. In this modality, individuals are taught to stand upright for 20 to 40 minutes a day in an effort to cause presyncope. In the athlete and young individual these nonpharmacologic approaches should initially be used with only those failing the more conservative measures. Pharmacological approaches to neurocardiogenic syncope have to this point only rarely been evaluated in randomized controlled trials, and in those trials they have generally been disappointing [46]. If pharmacologic therapy is necessary, the best data to support their use is with selective serotonin uptake inhibitors and midodrine [46]. Pacing therapy should be considered for those with particularly malignant syncope that has a marked negative chronotropic component (Fig. 1) [61]. Because neurocardiogenic syncope is not life threatening, and because it is unlikely to occur during exertion, athletes are not prevented from sporting activities.

Bradyarrhythmias

Bradyarrhythmias that cause syncope are generally acute in onset and can cause injury. However, bradycardia is common in the athlete, especially at rest, and rarely causes syncope. According to the Bethesda Conference guidelines, athletes with first degree or Mobitz I heart block, which does not worsen with exercise, do not need treatment or restriction of competitive athletics [6,62]. However, athletes with Mobitz II or complete heart block generally require pacing. Individuals with congenital heart block, while possessing an adequate escape early in life, will benefit from pacing as they age. Those athletes with permanent pacemakers should not participate in competitive athletics with a danger of bodily collision [6,62].

Supraventricular arrhythmias

Supraventricular arrhythmias rarely cause syncope and more commonly cause palpitations and lightheadedness (Fig. 2). Treatment of supraventricular arrhythmias can be accomplished with beta-blocking agents, calcium channel blocking agents, digoxin, antiarrhythmic agents, and ablative procedures. Beta-blockers can be effective in many patients; however, they are banned in some competitive sports and many young patients have intolerable side effects. Antiarrhythmic agents are effective in many supraventricular tachyarrhythmias, but concern about proarrhythmias and

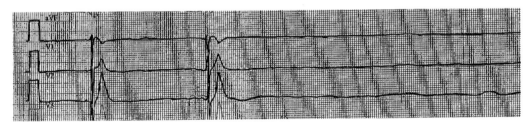

Fig. 1. Electrogram of a 23-year-old male in the recovery stage of a stress test. The patient had 13 episodes of exertional and postexertion syncope. During the recovery stage of the stress test he had a syncopal event and 30 seconds of asystole. A diagnosis of malignant neurocardiogenic syncope was made. A tilt-table test was also positive. Because of the profound asystole, he was treated with a permanent pacemaker.

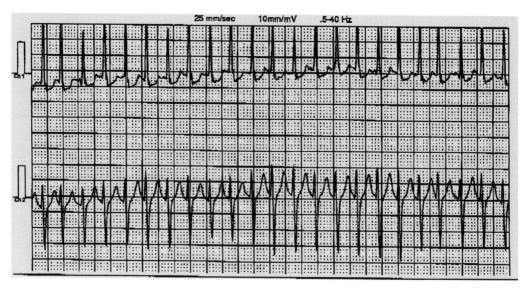

Fig. 2. Loop monitor recording of a 20-year-old female who, during basketball games, would have sudden onset of palpitations, lightheadedness, and fatigue, limiting but not eliminating her ability to play ball. Her coaches thought that she wasn't trying hard enough, until this loop monitor documented a narrow complex tachycardia that was the cause of her symptoms. At an invasive electrophysiologic evaluation she was found to have AV nodal reentrant tachycardia which was successfully ablated.

long-term use limit their use in this young patient cohort. The two most common supraventricular arrhythmias (AV nodal reentrant tachycardia and Wolff-Parkinson-White syndrome) are usually readily cured with radiofrequency ablation. This procedure can be accomplished with low morbidity, and in the young athlete radiofrequency ablation should be considered as initial treatment. According to the Bethesda Conference guidelines, athletes with radiofrequency cure of supraventricular tachycardias can resume competitive athletics after 4 weeks [6,62].

Ventricular arrhythmias

Ventricular arrhythmias typically cause acute syncope without preceding symptoms. Yet, some individuals will not have loss of consciousness, but palpitations and lightheadedness. These arrhythmias are most likely to occur during peak exertion. Only ventricular tachyarrhythmias associated with normal hearts are currently curable. In these patients without structural heart disease, cure rates with radiofrequency ablation approach 90%, with a low incidence of complications [63]. On the other hand, in patients with underlying structural heart disease, cure of the underlying disease and thus of their

predisposition to ventricular arrhythmias is unlikely. Radiofrequency ablation in ventricular arrhythmias in the presence of heart disease cannot be relied upon to protect against sudden death. According to the Bethesda Conference, only low intensity competitive athletics is permitted in athletes with structural heart disease and sustained ventricular arrhythmias, without regard to the method of treatment [62].

In the patient with hypertrophic cardiomyopathy, several strategies have been developed and include surgery, beta-blockers, antiarrhythmic agents, permanent pacemakers, and implantable cardioverter defibrillators (ICDs). Implantation of the ICD is the surest way to prevent sudden cardiac death (Fig. 3) [64]. In those athletes with hypertrophic cardiomyopathy that survive sudden death an ICD should be offered. In others thought to be at high risk based on family medical history of sudden death, personal history of syncope, massively thick septum, nonsustained ventricular tachycardia, or a hypotensive response to exercise, an ICD may be appropriate. In those patients with a lower risk of sudden death an ICD is an option, but not universally agreed upon. In most individuals with hypertrophic cardiomyopathy, competitive athletics should be prohibited and beta-blockers should be prescribed [65].

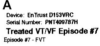

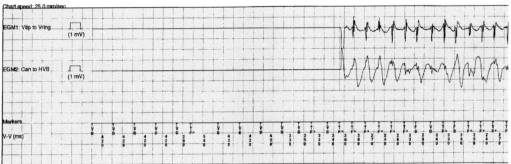

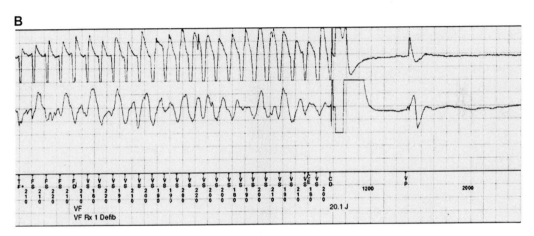

Fig. 3. Initiation (*A*) and termination (*B*) of ventricular fibrillation in a 9-year-old boy with hypertrophic cardiomyopathy and an ICD. He presented 3 months earlier with syncope during a school gym class and was found to have hypertrophic cardiomyopathy. Because of the syncope and hypertrophic cardiomyopathy, an ICD was recommended and placed. This current episode also caused syncope and the ICD promptly defibrillated him.

ARVD is likely a progressive disease; thus treatments effective at one point may become ineffective later in time [66]. Radiofrequency ablation is rarely curative [67]. Sotalol and amiodarone may decrease the frequency of arrhythmias. Current opinions of the optimal treatment of these patients vary, but in those of sufficiently high risk for sudden death an ICD should be considered [68]. Moderate and high level competitive athletics are contraindicated, in view of the frequent provocation of arrhythmias with exercise [6,62].

Patients with the long QT syndrome should be placed on beta-blockers. In those with recurrent syncope on beta-blockers, or those thought to be at high risk of SCD, an ICD is warranted [69–71]. Restriction from competitive sports is recommended for those with syncope or resuscitated SCD,

and for those with QTC above 470 in males and 480 in females [62].

In the individual with idiopathic cardiomyopathy, beta-blockers and angiotensin-converting enzyme inhibitors lower the risk of all cause mortality and sudden death and should be prescribed to all patients. Generally, individuals with idiopathic cardiomyopathy with left ventricular ejection fractions less than or equal to 35% should be treated with an ICD [72,73]. In patients with idiopathic cardiomyopathy and a prior spontaneous sustained ventricular arrhythmia, competitive athletics of moderate or high intensity should be avoided [6,62].

In patients with coronary artery disease and ventricular arrhythmias, ICDs offer the best protection against sudden death [74]. In addition, individuals with coronary artery disease and left ventricular ejection fractions less than or equal to 35%, an ICD should be offered [73,75]. In athletes with coronary artery disease and ventricular arrhythmias, only low intensity competitive athletics are permitted [6,62].

The Brugada syndrome, a specific genetic abnormality of the SCN5A channel, may cause syncope and sudden death in young individuals [76]. Individuals are diagnosed by abnormal 12-lead ECGs in which incomplete right bundle branch blocks and ST-segment elevations are seen in the precordial leads. Symptomatic patients (ie, syncope or resuscitated sudden death) with the Brugada syndrome should be treated with ICDs; however, the treatment of asymptomatic individuals with Brugada syndrome is controversial [76]. Because of the potential for SCD and the lack of data regarding exertion and Brugada Syndrome, for the current time competitive athletics are not recommended [62].

Summary

Athletes with syncope warrant a full evaluation. These athletes may suffer from neurocardiogenic syncope, the most common cause of syncope in the young. In this case their prognosis is excellent and they can continue to compete. However, it is also possible that athletics may unmask heart disease, either structural or electrical, and these athletes may be at risk of sudden cardiac death. The workup and treatment of syncope in the athlete offers some unique challenges: to diagnose potentially life-threatening arrhythmias, to avoid pharmacological therapy, and to maximize ability to play. Radiofrequency ablation should be offered to those athletes with conditions in which a cure is possible. Restriction of competitive athletics is necessary for those with life threatening conditions while those with benign conditions can continue to compete.

References

[1] Link MS, Homoud MK, Wang PJ, et al. Syncope in athletes. Cardiovasc Rev Rep 2002;23:625–32.
[2] Estes NA 3rd, Link MS, Cannom D, et al. Report of the NASPE policy conference on arrhythmias and the athlete. J Cardiovasc Electrophysiol 2001;12:1208–19.
[3] Kramer MR, Drori Y, Lev B. Sudden death in young soldiers: high incidence of syncope prior to death. Chest 1988;93:345–7.
[4] Maron BJ, Roberts WC, McAllister HA, et al. Sudden death in young athletes. Circulation 1980;62:218–29.
[5] Mitchell JH, Haskell W, Snell P, et al. Task Force 8: classification of sports. 36th Bethesda Conference: eligibility recommendations for competitive athletes with cardiovascular abnormalities. J Am Coll Cardiol 2005;45:1364–7.
[6] Murdoch BD. Loss of consciousness in healthy South African men: incidence, causes and relationship to EEG abnormality. S Afr Med J 1980;57:771–4.
[7] Colivicchi F, Ammirati F, Santini M. Epidemiology and prognostic implications of syncope in young competing athletes. Eur Heart J 2004;25:1749–53.
[8] Albert CM, Mittleman MA, Chae CU, et al, Triggering of sudden death from cardiac causes by vigorous exertion. N Engl J Med 2000;343:1355–61.
[9] Mittleman MA, MaClure M, Tofler GH, et al. Triggering of acute myocardial infarction by heavy physical exertion. N Engl J Med 1993;329:1677–83.
[10] Corrado D, Basso C, Rizzoli G, et al. Does sports activity enhance the risk of sudden death in adolescents and young adults? J Am Coll Cardiol 2003;42:1959–63.
[11] Corrado D, Migliore F, Basso C, et al. Exercise and the risk of sudden cardiac death. Herz 2006;31:553–8.
[12] Tofler GH. Triggers of sudden cardiac death in the athlete. In: Estes NAM, Salem DN, Wang PJ, editors. Sudden cardiac death in the athlete. Armonk (NY): Futura Publishing Company, Inc.; 1998. p. 221–34.
[13] Thompson PD. The Cardiovascular risks of exercise. In: Thompson PD, editor. Exercise and sports cardiology. New York: McGraw-Hill; 2001. p. 127–45.
[14] Strickberger SA, Benson DW, Biaggioni I, et al. AHA/ACCF Scientific Statement on the evaluation of syncope: from the American Heart Association Councils on Clinical Cardiology, Cardiovascular Nursing, Cardiovascular Disease in the Young, and Stroke, and the Quality of Care and Outcomes Research Interdisciplinary Working Group; and the American College of Cardiology Foundation: in collaboration with the Heart Rhythm Society: endorsed by the American Autonomic Society. Circulation 2006;113:316–27.
[15] Maron BJ. Sudden death in young athletes. N Engl J Med 2003;349:1064–75.
[16] Maron BJ, Pelliccia A. The heart of trained athletes: cardiac remodeling and the risks of sports, including sudden death. Circulation 2006;114:1633–44.
[17] Corrado D, Thiene G, Nava A, et al. Sudden death in young competitive athletes: clinicopathologic correlations in 22 cases. Am J Med 1990;89:588–96.
[18] Pelliccia A, Di Paolo FM, Corrado D, et al. Evidence for efficacy of the Italian national pre-participation screening programme for identification of hypertrophic cardiomyopathy in competitive athletes. Eur Heart J 2006;27:2196–200.

[19] Graham TP Jr, Driscoll DJ, Gersony WM, et al. Task Force 2: congenital heart disease. J Am Coll Cardiol 2005;45:1326–33.

[20] Maron BJ, Estes NA 3rd, Link MS. Task Force 11: Commotio cordis: 36th Bethesda Conference: Eligibility Recommendations for Competitive Athletes With Cardiovascular Abnormalities. J Am Coll Cardiol 2005;45:1371–3.

[21] Maron BJ, Gohman TE, Kyle SB, et al. Clinical profile and spectrum of commotio cordis. JAMA 2002;287:1142–6, 18.

[22] Calkins H, Shyr Y, Frumin H, et al. The value of the clinical history in the differentiation of syncope due to ventricular tachycardia, atrioventricular block, and neurocardiogenic syncope. Am J Med 1995;98: 365–73.

[23] Kapoor WN. Evaluation and outcome of patients with syncope. Medicine (Baltimore) 1990;69:160–75.

[24] Alboni P, Brignole M, Menozzi C, et al. Diagnostic value of history in patients with syncope with or without heart disease. J Am Coll Cardiol 2001;37: 1921–8.

[25] McGovern BA, Liberthson R. Arrhythmias induced by exercise in athletes and others. S Afr Med J 1996; 86:C78–82.

[26] Sneddon JF, Scalia G, Ward DE, et al. Exercise induced vasodepressor syncope. Br Heart J 1994; 71:554–7.

[27] Sakaguchi S, Shultz JJ, Remole SC, et al. Syncope associated with exercise, a manifestation of neurally mediated syncope. Am J Cardiol 1995;75:476–81.

[28] Calkins H, Siefert M, Morady F. Clinical presentation and long-term follow-up of athletes with exercise-induced vasodepressor syncope. Am Heart J 1995;129:1159–64.

[29] Kosinski D, Grubb BP, Kip K, et al. Exercise-induced neurocardiogenic syncope. Am Heart J 1996;132:451–2.

[30] Eichna LW, Horvath S, Bean WB. Post-exertional orthostatic hypotension. Am J Med Sci 1947;213: 641–54.

[31] Holtzhausen LM, Noakes TD. The prevalence and significance of post-exercise (postural) hypotension in ultramarathon runners. Med Sci Sports Exerc 1995;27:1595–601.

[32] Link MS, Wang PJ, Estes NA 3rd. Ventricular arrhythmias in the athlete. Curr Opin Cardiol 2001;16:30–9.

[33] Pelliccia A, Maron BJ, Culasso F, et al. Clinical significance of abnormal electrocardiographic patterns in trained athletes. Circulation 2000;102: 278–84.

[34] Serra-Grima R, Estorch M, Carrio I, et al. Marked ventricular repolarization abnormalities in highly trained athletes' electrocardiograms: clinical and prognostic implications. J Am Coll Cardiol 2000; 36:1310–6.

[35] Zehender M, Meinertz T, Keul J, et al. ECG variants and cardiac arrhythmias in athletes: clinical

relevance and prognostic importance. Am Heart J 1990;119:1378–91.

[36] Balady GJ, Cadigan JB, Ryan TJ. Electrocardiogram of the athlete: an analysis of 289 professional football players. Am J Cardiol 1984;53:1339–43.

[37] Oakley CM. The electrocardiogram in the highly trained athlete. Cardiol Clin 1992;10:295–302.

[38] Wang K, Asinger R, Hodges M. Electrocardiograms of Wolff-Parkinson-White syndrome simulating other conditions. Am Heart J 1996;132:152–5.

[39] Ott P, Marcus FI. Electrocardiographic markers of sudden death. Cardiol Clin 2006;24:453–69, x.

[40] Nasir K, Bomma C, Tandri H, et al. Electrocardiographic features of arrhythmogenic right ventricular dysplasia/cardiomyopathy according to disease severity: a need to broaden diagnostic criteria. Circulation 2004;110:1527–34.

[41] Zareba W. Genotype-specific ECG patterns in long QT syndrome. J Electrocardiol 2006;39:S101–6.

[42] Moss AJ, Kass RS. Long QT syndrome: from channels to cardiac arrhythmias. J Clin Invest 2005;115: 2018–24.

[43] Schwartz PJ, Priori SG, Spazzolini C, et al. Genotype-phenotype correlation in the long-QT syndrome: gene-specific triggers for life-threatening arrhythmias. Circulation 2001;103:89–95.

[44] Benditt DG, Ferguson DW, Grubb BP, et al. ACC Expert Consensus Document: Tilt table testing for assessing syncope. J Am Coll Cardiol 1996;28: 263–75.

[45] Grubb BP, Temesy-Armos PN, Samoil D, et al. Tilt table testing in the evaluation and management of athletes with recurrent exercise-induced syncope. Med Sci Sports Exerc 1993;25:24–8.

[46] Grubb BP. Clinical practice. Neurocardiogenic syncope. N Engl J Med 2005;352:1004–10.

[47] Link MS, Estes NAM III. Ventricular arrhythmias. In: Estes NAM, Salem DN, Wang PJ, editors. Sudden cardiac death in the athlete. Armonk (NY): Futura Publishing Co., Inc.; 1998. p. 253–75.

[48] Klein GJ, Bashore TM, Sellers TD, et al. Ventricular fibrillation in the Wolff-Parkinson-White Syndrome. N Engl J Med 1979;301:1080–5.

[49] Leitch JW, Klein GJ, Yee R, et al. Prognostic value of electrophysiologic testing in asymptomatic patients with Wolff-Parkinson-White pattern. Circulation 1990;82:1718–23.

[50] Pappone C, Santinelli V. Should catheter ablation be performed in asymptomatic patients with Wolff-Parkinson-White syndrome? Catheter ablation should be performed in asymptomatic patients with Wolff-Parkinson-White syndrome. Circulation 2005;112:2207–15 [discussion: 2216].

[51] Wellens HJ. Should catheter ablation be performed in asymptomatic patients with Wolff-Parkinson-White syndrome? When to perform catheter ablation in asymptomatic patients with a Wolff-Parkinson-White electrocardiogram. Circulation 2005;112:2201–7 [discussion: 2216].

[52] Brugada P, Green M, Abdollah H, et al. Significance of ventricular arrhythmias initiated by programmed ventricular stimulation: the importance of the type of ventricular arrhythmia induced and the number of premature stimuli required. Circulation 1984;69: 87–92.

[53] Bigger JT, Reiffel JA, Livelli FD, et al. Sensitivity, specificity, and reproducibility of programmed ventricular stimulation. Circulation 1986;73(suppl II): II73–8.

[54] Prystowsky EN. Electrophysiologic-electropharmacologic testing in patients with ventricular arrhythmias. Pacing Clin Electrophysiol 1988;11:225–51.

[55] Peters S, Reil GH. Risk factors of cardiac arrest in arrhythmogenic right ventricular dysplasia. Eur Heart J 1995;16:77–80.

[56] Corrado D, Leoni L, Calkins H, et al. Prophylactic implantable defibrillator in patients with arrhythmogenic right ventricular cardiomyopathy/dysplasia and no prior sustained ventricular tachyarrhythmias: therapy-based risk stratification during a long term follow-up. Circulation 2006:2006 Annual Scientific Sessions.

[57] Link MS, Homoud MK, Wang PJ, et al. Cardiac arrhythmias in the athlete: the evolving role of electrophysiology. Curr Sports Med Rep 2002;1: 75–85.

[58] Grubb BP, Kanjwal Y, Kosinski DJ. The postural tachycardia syndrome: a concise guide to diagnosis and management. J Cardiovasc Electrophysiol 2006;17:108–12.

[59] Grubb BP, Kosinski DJ, Kanjwal Y. Orthostatic hypotension: causes, classification, and treatment. Pacing Clin Electrophysiol 2003;26:892–901.

[60] DiGirolamo E, Di Iorio C, Leonzio L, et al. Usefulness of a tilt training program for the prevention of refractory neurocardiogenic syncope in adolescents: a controlled study. Circulation 1999;100:1798–801.

[61] Trim GM, Krahn AD, Klein GJ, et al. Pacing for vasovagal syncope after the second Vasovagal Pacemaker Study (VPS II): a matter of judgement. Card Electrophysiol Rev 2003;7:416–20.

[62] Zipes DP, Ackerman MJ, Estes NAM III, et al. Task Force 7: arrhythmias. 36th Bethesda Conference: eligibility recommendations for competitive athletes with cardiovascular abnormalities. J Am Coll Cardiol 2005;45:43–52.

[63] Stevenson WG. Catheter ablation of monomorphic ventricular tachycardia. Curr Opin Cardiol 2005; 20:42–7.

[64] Maron BJ, Shen WK, Link MS, et al. Efficacy of the implantable cardioverter-defibrillator for the prevention of sudden death in patients with hypertrophic cardiomyopathy. N Engl J Med 2000;342: 365–73.

[65] Maron BJ, Ackerman MJ, Nishimura RA, et al. Task Force 4: HCM and other cardiomyopathies, mitral valve prolapse, myocarditis, and Marfan syndrome. 36th Bethesda Conference: Eligibility Recommendations for Competitive Athletes With Cardiovascular Abnormalities. J Am Coll Cardiol 2005;45:1340–5.

[66] Corrado D, Basso C, Thiene G, et al. Spectrum of clinicopathologic manifestations of arrhythmogenic right ventricular cardiomyopathy/dysplasia: a multicenter study. J Am Coll Cardiol 1997;30:1512–20.

[67] Shoda M, Kasanuki H, Ohnishi S, et al. Recurrence of new ventricular tachycardia after successful catheter ablation in patients with arrhythmogenic right ventricular dysplasia. Circulation 1992;86:I-580.

[68] Corrado D, Leoni L, Link MS, et al. Implantable cardioverter-defibrillator therapy for prevention of sudden death in patients with arrhythmogenic right ventricular cardiomyopathy/dysplasia. Circulation 2003;108:3084–91.

[69] Moss AJ, Zareba W, Hall WJ, et al. Effectiveness and limitations of beta-blocker therapy in congenital long-QT syndrome. Circulation 2000;101:616–23.

[70] Hobbs JB, Peterson DR, Moss AJ, et al. Risk of aborted cardiac arrest or sudden cardiac death during adolescence in the long-QT syndrome. JAMA 2006;296:1249–54.

[71] Sauer AJ, Moss AJ, McNitt S, et al. Long QT syndrome in adults. J Am Coll Cardiol 2007;49:329–37.

[72] Kadish A, Dyer A, Daubert JP, et al. Prophylactic defibrillator implantation in patients with nonischemic dilated cardiomyopathy. N Engl J Med 2004; 350:2151–8.

[73] Bardy GH, Lee KL, Mark DB, et al. Amiodarone or an implantable cardioverter-defibrillator for congestive heart failure. N Engl J Med 2005;352:225–37.

[74] AVID Investigators. A comparison of antiarrhythmic-drug therapy with implantable defibrillators in patients resuscitated from near-fatal ventricular arrhythmias. N Engl J Med 1997;337:1576–83.

[75] Moss AJ, Zareba W, Hall WJ, et al. Prophylactic implantation of a defibrillator in patients with myocardial infarction and reduced ejection fraction. N Engl J Med 2002;346:877–83.

[76] Antzelevitch C, Brugada P, Borggrefe M, et al. Brugada syndrome: report of the second consensus conference: endorsed by the Heart Rhythm Society and the European Heart Rhythm Association. Circulation 2005;111:659–70.

Implantable Cardioverter Defibrillator Therapy in Athletes

Hein Heidbüchel, MD, PhD

Cardiology–Electrophysiology, University Hospital Gasthuisberg, University of Leuven, Herestraat 49, B-3000 Leuven, Belgium, Europe

Over the last decade implantable cardioverter defibrillators (ICD) have become accepted therapy in patients with ventricular arrhythmias. They can be used for secondary prophylaxis, such as after a prior cardiac arrest caused by ventricular fibrillation (VF), or in patients who have developed a sustained ventricular tachycardia (VT) with hemodynamic compromise. They are also used progressively more often for primary prophylactic indications, as in patients with left ventricular systolic dysfunction or inherited cardiomyopathies with increased risk for sudden death. Also, in athletic and physically active young people, ICDs can be applied for secondary or primary prophylaxis. Their use in this patient group, however, implies some specific considerations, which form the subject of this article.

Indications for ICD therapy in athletes

The indications for ICD therapy in general have been extensively reviewed in recently updated American College of Cardiology/American Heart Association Task Force and the European Society of Cardiology guidelines on the management of patients with ventricular arrhythmia [1]. Their use in athletes has also been outlined in North American and European guidelines [2–4].

More recent recommendations have described ICD indications in patients performing leisure time physical activity [5].

In most athletes treated with an ICD, underlying structural heart disease or an inherited channelopathy (like the long QT syndrome) is present. However, this underlying etiology may not have been overt before. Intensive exertion may trigger ventricular arrhythmias at a time when no other symptoms of the underlying pathology are obvious. Therefore, documented ventricular arrhythmias during regular follow-up of athletes, or revealed after more thorough cardiovascular evaluation for aspecific symptoms (such as exertional dizziness, shortness of breath, or syncope), should prompt a careful assessment. Long-term ECG recordings (by Holter or event recorder) may show frequent ventricular ectopy or nonsustained ventricular tachycardia. Imaging techniques such as echocardiography, cardiac magnetic resonance imaging, nuclear scintigraphy, or coronary angiography may reveal underlying dilated, hypertrophic or right ventricular cardiomyopathy, valve disease, or atherosclerotic heart disease. Further electrophysiological workup is often required, and can include a signal averaged ECG (to detect late potentials) or even an invasive electrophysiological study in some. In addition, the baseline ECG may reveal important underlying causes (hypertrophic cardiomyopathy, arrhythmogenic right ventricular cardiomyopathy, long QT syndrome, short QT syndrome, or Brugada-syndrome) and has therefore been recommended as part of regular screening of athletes [6]. When no causal therapy is available to prevent arrhythmia recurrences (as is often the case), and when the risk of a potentially life-threatening

The author receives an unconditional research grant for the Electrophysiology Section of the Cardiology Department of the University Hospital Gasthuisberg from Medtronic.

Hein Heidbüchel is holder of the AstraZeneca Chair in Cardiology, University of Leuven.

E-mail address: hein.heidbuchel@uz.kuleuven.ac.be

arrhythmia is estimated to be high, implantation of an ICD is warranted.

Because of more widespread screening in family members with inherited arrhythmogenic conditions (channelopathies or cardiomyopathies) and the rapid progress in genotypic identification of silent mutation carriers, the group of young and physically active patients eligible for primary ICD implantation is rapidly growing. The rationale for this is that the first symptomatic manifestation of the hereditary disease may be sudden death, and that exertion often plays a triggering role.

Device selection and implantation

For detection of life-threatening ventricular arrhythmias, ICDs rely mainly on the rate information of a right ventricular (RV) electrode. In many patients, implantation is performed with only a single RV lead (single-chamber ICD or VVI-ICD). Different rate zones can be programmed and therapies specified for these different zones. For the fastest rate, considered as the VF-rate zone by the ICD, shock therapy is programmed (and in some modern devices a single antitachypacing protocol during charging of the ICD). While in many elderly ICD recipients the threshold for this VF zone may be around 180 beats per minute (bpm), the active lifestyle of younger patients may require elevation of the threshold to more than 200 bpm. Accurate detection of fast ventricular rates depends on good sensing signals, which are of even more importance in this patient population and should be critically assessed during lead implantation.

Most devices can deliver a maximal energy of 30 J to 35 J to terminate VF. Although defibrillation can usually be achieved with 8 J to 12 J (defibrillation threshold), a safety margin of at least 10 J has to be programmed; therefore, during implantation the defibrillation threshold is determined. Shocks of more than a few joules are always painful. Hence, programming of the ICD will aim to prevent shocks by programming antitachycardia pacing whenever possible for slower and regular rates (VT zones). A train of pacing stimuli, well timed in relation to the spontaneous arrhythmia, is able to terminate the arrhythmia in an almost asymptomatic way in many patients. Electrophysiologic evaluation before implantation can help to determine the rate and type of spontaneous or inducible arrhythmias and whether they are pace-terminable or not.

It has been shown that even for ventricular rates up to 250 bpm, empirical programming of rapid antitachypacing may lead to arrhythmia termination in 72% [7].

When slower VTs are present, their detection may overlap with the sinus rates during exertion in young active patients. Therefore, additional discrimination between VT and sinus tachycardia may be required to prevent inappropriate antitachypacing or shocks. Some have advocated the implantation of a dual chamber ICD (ie, with an atrial plus a ventricular lead or DDD-ICD) in such cases, with the expectation that atrial electrogram information may increase the specificity of arrhythmia detection. However, this is rarely relevant in athletic patients. Even when they present with slow VT (which is less prevalent than in the more general coronary heart disease ICD population), these VTs may develop during exertion and sinus tachycardia. This may lead to inappropriate withholding of therapy (ie, decreased specificity). Moreover, dual chamber algorithms in modern ICD will opt to deliver ventricular therapy irrespective of the observed atrial rate in most cases (Fig. 1). Studies have shown that DDD-ICDs do not lead to a significant decreased incidence of inappropriate ICD therapy versus VVI-devices [8,9]. The algorithms based on comparison of atrial and ventricular rates and timing intervals are very complex, are different among different ICD manufactures, and are currently largely inaccessible for programming by the physicians (black box design). Although some smaller studies have suggested superiority of one algorithm over another, no large-scale prospective trials are available, although one is ongoing [10]. Therefore, at present no formal recommendations can be given on which DDD-device would be best suited in an athletic population. However, there may be other indications as to when to opt for a dual chamber ICD:

Rare patients may have a concomitant bradyarrhythmia indication, although sinus bradycardia is physiologic in most athletes and atrioventricular (AV) block is very rare.
When bradycardic agents are needed for prevention of inappropriate shocks (as discussed below), symptomatic bradycardia could be anticipated.
Atrial pacing may prevent atrial or ventricular arrhythmias, as in patients with concomitant atrial fibrillation and especially in patients with the long QT syndrome.

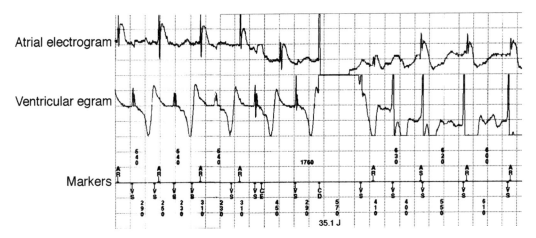

Fig. 1. Inappropriate shock delivery by a DDD-ICD despite sinus rhythm detection on the atrial lead. This young patient developed T-wave oversensing and double counting during moderate physical activity and with a sinus rate of 110/min. Despite unambiguous sensing of this sinus rhythm in the atrial channel, the fast mean ventricular rate led to (inappropriate) detection of VF and shock delivery (in the T-wave, with induction of a nonsustained slow ventricular arrhythmia).

Some patients with hypertrophic obstructive cardiomyopathy may have lower outflow gradients during AV sequential pacing with short AV intervals.

An extra atrial lead to the defibrillator configuration adds complexity during implant and follow-up. Large trials have clearly shown a higher incidence of early and late postoperative complications in dual-chamber devices [11]. This is an especially important consideration in a young patient group, such as athletes. No data are available for long-term follow-up, but many patients will require replacement of the original ventricular ICD lead. Ventricular ICD leads are much more complex than traditional pacing leads (because of additional conductors for one or two shock coils and the high voltages delivered) and may fail after 5 to 15 years [12,13]. Multiple leads may also result in subclavian vein thrombosis. If fewer leads are implanted during the initial procedure at a young age, extraction or placement of additional leads will be less indicated and less complicated, thus reducing morbidity (and mortality) in the longer term. All these considerations should be carefully weighted when selecting the proper ICD device for implantation in a young athletic patient. The above argument indicates that in many young patients a simple VVI-device may suffice, unless there are specific reasons for implantation of an atrial lead.

Finally, cardiac resynchronization therapy (CRT) ICDs (ie, devices with a third left ventricular electrode in addition to an atrial and right ventricular electrode) have no indication in physically active or athletic patients. They are implanted in patients with symptoms of heart failure which, because of this clinical situation, prohibits moderate to intense recreational or competitive sports. There may be a trend during the coming years to implant CRT devices at earlier stages of left ventricular dysfunction (ie, before heart failure symptoms emerge). Moreover, patients with CRT-ICD often participate in rehabilitation programs and recreational sports activity.

Since the ICD housing—or can—acts as one of the electrodes to defibrillate the heart with high-voltage shocks, implantation of an ICD needs to be mandatory at the left infraclavicular region so that the heart is located between the can and the RV shock coil. To prevent lead fracture, extreme ipsilateral arm movements should be avoided, such as during volleyball, basketball, tennis, racket sports, handball, swimming, gymnastics, or ballet. Moreover, such movements could result in lead dislocation, mainly during the first 6 weeks after implant but also later. Patients should therefore be instructed not to elevate their left arm above shoulder level during these first 6 weeks. This may lead to specific sports participation restrictions. In patients with left arm dominance (like left-handed tennis players) there is a higher risk for lead fracture caused by costo-clavicular crush. An example of a partial lead fracture is shown in Fig. 2. Although there are reports about adequate defibrillation with right-sided implanted defibrillators, such an approach cannot be advocated as standard practice. Most devices now allow noninvasive evaluation of the shock coil impedance, obviating the need for regular chest X-rays to detect lead fracture. The risk of subclavian crush, which is higher in all physically active patients but especially left-handed athletes, should be another impetus for implanting single-lead devices or VVI-ICD, and with a lead which is as simple as possible (ie, with minimal conductors, thus preferably with only one shocking coil) whenever feasible.

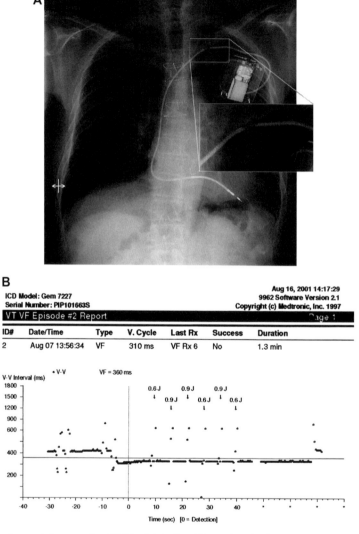

Fig. 2. Costo-clavicular crush fracture of an ICD lead. (*A*) Chest X-ray, showing fracture of the high voltage conductor in the ICD lead at the costo-clavicular junction. The broken helical conductor connected to the ventricular shock coil. The inner conductors of the pacing/sensing bipole were intact. (*B*) The fracture resulted in nondelivery of shocks during an episode of ventricular tachycardia despite correct detection. Although all therapies in this VF-rate zone had been programmed to 30 J, less than 1 J could be delivered. Like all ICDs, the device stopped delivering therapies after six unsuccessful shocks. Luckily for the patient, the arrhythmia terminated spontaneously after 1.3 minutes (right side of the figure).

Device programming

The programming of rate zones and zone-dependent therapies has been discussed before. Apart from atrial electrograms (requiring a DDD-ICD), detection algorithms may include other parameters to make VT identification more specific. Most ICDs allow programming of a sudden onset parameter, which sets a threshold value for change in rate to differentiate sinus tachycardia from ventricular arrhythmias. However, one should be cautious about using this parameter in physically active patients as ventricular arrhythmias may develop during sinus tachycardia, reducing the specificity of this discriminator. It can, however, be programmed in combination with an extended high rate parameter: even when sudden onset was not met, an arrhythmia persisting longer than the set time will trigger ICD interventions.

Many current ICD devices also have waveform discrimination algorithms that compare the morphology of QRS complexes during tachycardia with those during sinus rhythm. An example of such an algorithm, correctly rejecting a paroxysmal tachycardia as "supraventricular," is shown in Fig. 3. Another example from a different manufacturer, with correct classification of a wide QRS tachycardia as VT (and successful termination by ramp pacing) is shown in Fig. 4.

One needs to realize that all algorithms that increase the specificity of arrhythmia discrimination may also lead to decreased sensitivity, that is, possible rejection of appropriate detection of VT. It is clear that nondetection of a ventricular arrhythmia can have serious consequences. Many electrophysiologists therefore will opt not to program these discriminators on unless there are particular indications, such as after inappropriate shock delivery. Modern devices provide feedback on how they would have classified an arrhythmia if detection discriminators had been programmed on. In such circumstances, it may be warranted to increase the detection specificity.

Programming of the bradycardia pacing function of the ICD in athletes can usually be done at a very low backup rate: most have no bradycardia pacing indication, and ventricular pacing by itself may be symptomatic. As outlined above, pacing for symptomatic bradycardia is rarely an indication in young active ICD recipients. However, some patients may have chronotropic incompetence, while in others it may be anticipated that bradycardic agents, required to prevent rapid conduction of supraventricular tachycardia, could lead to symptomatic bradycardia at rest. AV sequential pacing in such circumstances prevents symptoms caused by sole ventricular pacing. If rate responsiveness is required, appropriate rate acceleration during the particular sport activity of the athlete needs to be evaluated. This can be done by performing long-term ECG recording during these activities. Conversely, inappropriate rate acceleration during sports participation needs to be excluded.

An example has been published about inappropriate accelerometer activation during horseback riding [14]. Although pacemakers with dual sensors (minute ventilation plus activity) have been shown to be able to better adapt to different loads [15], dual sensors are not available in defibrillators. Moreover, the upper rate limit of rate responsive pacing in ICD patients is usually restricted by the requirement to detect ventricular arrhythmias, preventing programming of high pacing rates. An adaptive AV delay may help to increase the upper rate limit but may increase the degree of right ventricular pacing. On the other hand, in most patients with ICDs it is recommended to refrain from moderate and intensive physical activity, which obviates the need for high upper rate limits.

Recommendations on sports participation in ICD patients

General recommendations

The underlying pathological conditions that lead to ICD implantation usually require limitations in sports participation. Generally, they include the advice to abstain from intensive sports or competitive participation. Although very effective in preventing sudden death, ICD implantation should not be regarded as a substitute for such a recommendation [16]. Moreover, there are other reasons to abstain from intensive sports participation with an ICD: (1) physical activity is a likely trigger for ventricular arrhythmias, that can be better prevented than treated; (2) transient impaired consciousness can have far-reaching implications during certain sports; and (3) the efficacy of the ICD to interrupt malignant ventricular arrhythmias during intense exercise is unknown and, from theoretical considerations, probably suboptimal (given the associated metabolic, autonomic, and potentially ischemic conditions).

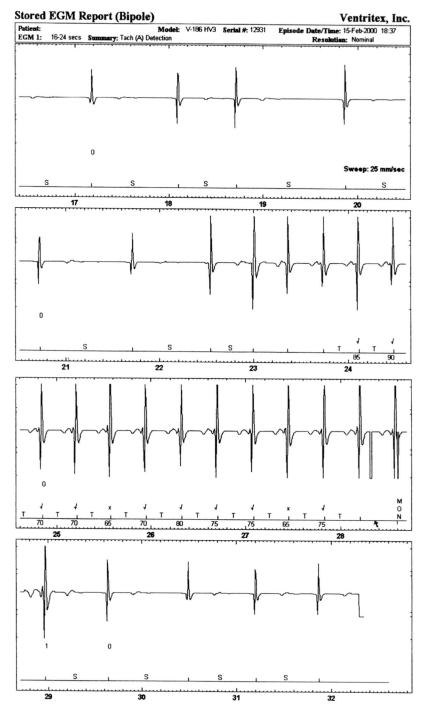

Fig. 3. Morphology discrimination of arrhythmia. The four panels show consecutive intracardiac electrograms recorded by an ICD during arrhythmia detection. Although there was a sudden onset (ie, sudden increase of the ventricular rate into the VT-rate zone), the electrogram morphology matched that of the intracardiac QRS-complex during the foregoing atrial fibrillation rhythm (as indicated by the check marks at the bottom of the tracings). This resulted in declassification of VT detection by the device and thus withholding of inappropriate therapy.

A

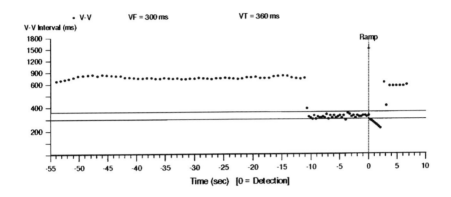

ICD Model: Gem 7227
Serial Number: PIP105378S

Feb 18, 2002 14:43:11
9962 Software Version 4.0
Copyright Medtronic, Inc. 2000

VT/VF Episode #6 Report

Page 1

ID#	Date/Time	Type	V. Cycle	Last Rx	Success	Duration
6	Feb 18 04:41:07	VT	320 ms	VT Rx 1	Yes	12 sec

B

ICD Model: Gem 7227
Serial Number: PIP105378S

Feb 18, 2002 14:43:18
9962 Software Version 4.0
Copyright Medtronic, Inc. 2000

VT/VF Episode #6 Report

Page 1

ID#	Date/Time	Type	V. Cycle	Last Rx	Success	Duration
6	Feb 18 04:41:07	VT	320 ms	VT Rx 1	Yes	12 sec

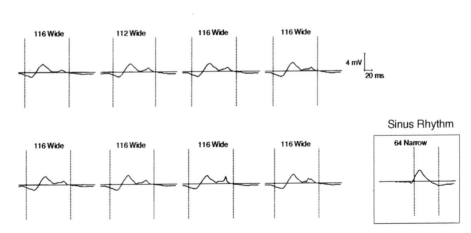

Fig. 4. Morphology discrimination of arrhythmia. (*A*) Interval plot showing how an arrhythmia suddenly started during sinus rhythm of about 70 bpm (V-V interval 800 ms): the ventricular rate accelerated to 188 bpm (320 ms). In this VT zone, morphology discrimination had been activated. (*B*) The width of eight consecutive beats was compared with a previously stored template during sinus rhythm (right lower corner; not normal part of the printout but added for didactical clarity). It was wider in all beats (112 ms or 116 ms versus 64 ms). The arrhythmia was correctly classified as ventricular tachycardia, and ramp antitachypacing was delivered resulting in termination of VT with resumption of sinus rhythm (see right side of Fig. *A*).

Therefore, an ICD disqualifies an athlete for competitive sports, except those with a low cardiovascular demand (such as golf, billiards, or bowling) [4,17]. However, physicians and patients alike may feel more assured to continue leisure-time physical activities with low to moderate dynamic or static demand (and without risk of bodily collision) with an ICD on board, which may contribute to physical and psychologic well-being [18]. Specific data on the benefits and risks of ICD in physically active patients are lacking, explaining a large variability in current recommendations made by physicians to their patients [19]. Some physicians have opted to allow competitive sports in particular cases. In a survey of Heart Rhythm Society members, ICD shocks were common during sports, but injury to the patient and to the ICD system were relatively rare (less than 1% and 5%, respectively) [19]. There were, however, two reported deaths, one because of head injuries caused by a fall. Further data are certainly needed to better define levels of sports participation with acceptable risk.

The device itself is an important monitor of physiologic heart rates, (nonsustained) arrhythmias, and the sinus rate at which ventricular arrhythmias occur. A specific monitoring zone, with detection but without therapies, can be specifically programmed for this purpose. After a period without problems (6 months, 1 year, or longer), the level of participation can be adjusted and tailored to a target heart rate, which can be monitored on a wrist device by the patient. However, in patients with arrhythmias that are particularly sensitive to triggering by exercise, these recommendations should be made with caution.

Leisure-time sports resumption is allowed from 6 weeks after implant, preferably after a control stress test. When appropriate or inappropriate ICD interventions occur (antitachypacing or shocks), a 6-week period refraining from sports should be reconsidered to evaluate the effect of changes in medical therapy or ICD programming.

Type of sports

Sports participation with bodily contact is contra-indicated, given the risk for trauma to the subcutaneously implanted device and its connection with the lead system [20–24]. Therefore, sports like rugby, martial arts, shooting, or American football may have additional risks. Some have advocated padding of the ICD

implantation site, as designed for soccer, basketball, baseball, or hockey, although the effectiveness of these protection systems has never been proven.

Given the fact that there is latency between arrhythmia onset and ICD intervention to terminate it (by antitachypacing or shocks), sports activities during which dizziness or (pre)syncope would expose the patient or others to additional risks are relatively contra-indicated. Examples are climbing, piloting, and diving, among others.

Electromagnetic interference with ICD function is extremely rare. However, the patient should be instructed about this potentiality if encountering any sports-related exposition to electromagnetic fields, and ICD follow-up should explicitly exclude inappropriate detection. Strong magnetic fields could temporarily (or in certain models permanently) inhibit tachy-arrhythmia therapy, although no specific sports-related circumstances in which this has occurred have been described.

Inappropriate shocks

The most important clinical concern in athletic patients with implanted defibrillators is the delivery of inappropriate shocks. Because these shocks are painful, they may result in important psychological coping problems that can range from anxiety to aversion of the ICD therapy. Some athletes may even ask for explantation of the ICD out of fear of more inappropriate shocks. In addition, such shocks can be potentially life threatening because they may trigger malignant arrhythmias (Fig. 5) [25,26]. Inappropriate shocks occur in 16% to 44% of patients after 1 to 5 years of follow-up [8,27,28]. Surprisingly, the recent survey of Heart Rhythm Society members about ICD therapy during sports did not distinguish between appropriate or inappropriate therapies, although ICD shocks were reported to be common during sports [19].

Causes for inappropriate therapy delivery

The main reasons for inappropriate therapy delivery are supraventricular arrhythmias with rates into the VT or VF detection zone. In young and active patients this is often caused by sinus tachycardia. In addition, rapidly conducted atrial fibrillation or other atrial arrhythmias may trigger inappropriate shocks.

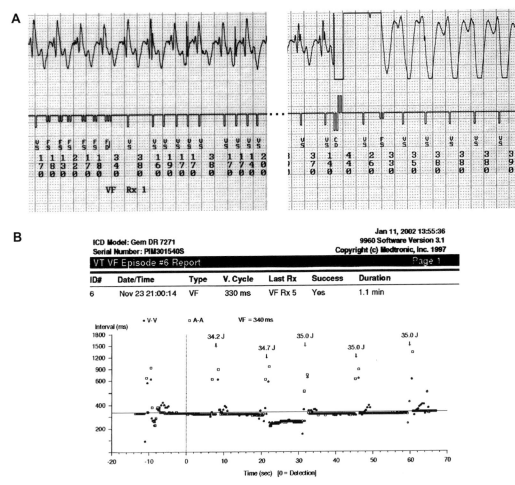

Fig. 5. Inappropriate shocks can be life threatening. (*A*) During exercising at a sinus rate of 170 bpm, this patient with Brugada syndrome developed large T-waves on his intracardiac sensing electrogram, resulting in counting of both R- and T-waves. The ICD interpreted the double rate of 340 bpm as ventricular fibrillation and delivered a shock of 24 J on the T-wave (CD in right panel). This shock induced real ventricular tachycardia at a rate of 160 bpm, which was later converted, with a shock of 30 J. (*B*) A similar proarrhythmic event occurred in another athlete in whom VF detection was triggered by sinus tachycardia of more than 180 bpm (see gradual decrease of R-R interval crossing the detection threshold of 330 ms). The time of detection is indicated by the vertical dotted line. A first shock of 35 J evidently did not modify the sinus tachycardia (with VF reconfirmation), but the second shock induced a real fast ventricular tachycardia of about 280 bpm (220 ms), which was converted back to sinus tachycardia by the third shock. Fortunately, two further shocks did not reinduce ventricular arrhythmia. The sinus rate gradually declined (the patient stopped his exertion), so that there was no further inappropriate detection after shock five. If the last shock (sixth to eighth) of such a consecutive series of inappropriate shocks would induce a ventricular arrhythmia, the device would not deliver further shocks, which evidently would lead to a life-threatening situation.

Other causes can be divided between intrinsic or extrinsic events, dependent on whether cardiac or extracardiac signals lead to inappropriate detection. Intrinsic events include far-field oversensing of atrial activity, as has been reported in ICDs with integrated bipolar sensing and a shock coil which extends into the right atrium [29]. Repetitive nonsustained ventricular tachycardia, or ventricular premature beats, may also lead to arrhythmia detection and delivery of shocks which in essence are not necessary [30]. The most common intrinsic reason for inappropriate detection is double counting of ventricular events caused by T-wave oversensing (Figs. 1, 5): every heart beat is then counted twice, which may lead to inappropriate detection during modest sinus tachycardia. This phenomenon is more frequently observed in Brugada syndrome or short QT syndrome [29,31], which are part of the indications for prophylactic ICD implantation in young patients. These syndromes may be associated with dynamic changes in the size of the R and T wave sensed by the ventricular lead. Integrated bipolar leads may also increase these incidents [29]. One should therefore be critical on the quality of the intracardiac electrograms during implantation, with a high R/T ratio.

Extrinsic causes of inappropriate detection can be diaphragmatic potentials, bad connections caused by loose setscrews or lead pins that are not fitted correctly within the defibrillator header, and electromagnetic interference (EMI). EMI is less frequent than anticipated because of the narrow band pass filters in modern devices; however, it remains an unpredictable cause of inappropriate detection. It has been described in association with the use of transcutaneous nerve stimulation [32], electrocautery [33], security gates, toys, washing machines, fish bond gear, and MRI equipment [34–37]. Although electrical and electronic environments during athletic participation could theoretically predispose to this complication, no case reports have described such interference. It should, however, be ruled out in case of athletes presenting with inappropriate shocks in specific locations. The most common extrinsic cause of inappropriate detections are lead problems, caused by insulation defect, abrasion, or fracture of the lead. An example is shown in Fig. 6. Insulation defects have been described in 4% to 22% of ICD patients after 4 to 6 years [13]. Prior device replacement is a risk factor for this complication [12,38,39]. Diagnosis requires evaluation of the electrograms during detection. Typically, these artifacts are exacerbated after high energy DC shock delivery, which leads to repetitive inappropriate shocks (see Fig. 6B, C). Other follow-up ICD parameters usually are normal in such situations (pacing threshold and impedance, shock impedance, battery voltage, and capacitor charge time), and often the bipolar sensing electrogram can return to perfectly normal tracings intermittently (and hence be missed during routine follow-up).

Acute management of inappropriate shocks

Most ICDs will stop firing after the delivery of six to eight shocks, considering an episode without success after such a series as untreatable or

inappropriately treated. This saves the patient with inappropriate detection from more shocks, although after a period that is considered as a sinus rhythm by the device, a new shock cluster may restart. Patients sometimes enter the hospital after having received multiple shocks. Therefore if a patient presents with an ICD shock or repetitive shocks (termed an "electrical storm") a thorough investigation is required into its cause. Of course, repetitive shocks can also be appropriate (VT or VF storm), although this is less common than clustered inappropriate shocks. It is important that when a patient enters an emergency ward for inappropriate shocks (and may be temporarily saved from further shocks by magnet application, see below), a 12-lead ECG and telemetric monitoring are obtained as soon as possible. Correct identification of the cause is key to preventing further shocks. If the ICD is interrogated to evaluate the cause of (inappropriate) therapy, one should make sure that the information is completely printed out and the ICD memory not erased, which could preclude further diagnostic evaluation.

It is advisable to put the patient immediately on telemetric ECG recording. If inappropriate shocks are delivered, they can be stopped by application of a magnet over the ICD. Generally, doughnut-shaped specific magnets are used, but also regular pacemaker magnets inhibit ICD function (Fig. 7). The magnet behavior is somewhat different depending on manufacturer. One should try to obtain information on the implanted device and the magnet response of it. An overview of magnet behavior is given in Table 1. Application of a magnet will, in almost any ICD, inhibit tachycardia therapy delivery while leaving bradycardia pacing unaffected (in Sorin/Ela Medical devices bradycardia pacing will be delivered at the magnet rate, which is dependent on the residual battery voltage). Usually, tachycardia detection is suspended, except in Boston Scientific (formerly Guidant) ICDs in which magnet application puts the device in a temporary "monitoring-only" mode (ie, detection of tachyarrhythmia but no automatic intervention). Older Guidant devices were also permanently deactivated if the magnet application lasted for more than 30 seconds. Although this is still a programmable option in modern Guidant ICDs, the default setting is a temporary inhibition, as in ICDs from other manufacturers. This means that if a real ventricular arrhythmia occurs and therapy delivery is necessary, the magnet can be removed with instantaneous resumption of full ICD function.

In most devices, interrogation of the ICD is possible while a magnet is applied (or a magnet is even obligatory in Biotronik and Medtronic ICDs). However, St. Jude and Sorin/Ela Medical devices cannot be interrogated while a magnet is in place, which can occasionally lead to an inability to reprogram the device during incessant tachycardia without letting the arrhythmia trigger another intervention. A printout of the electrograms that led to arrhythmia detection and therapy is of key importance in identifying its cause. (see Figs. 1, 3–6). Other parameters, such as pacing and shock lead impedance, can be helpful, as well as the amplitude and morphology of the sensed electrograms in sinus rhythm. Chest X-ray may reveal lead fracture or dislocation (see Fig. 2). Modern devices now measure some important device and lead related parameters (like lead impedance, sensing threshold and others) daily. A few devices have special counters that enable detection of artifactual potentials, based on unphysiologically short R-R intervals of less than 62 milleseconds in Sorin/Ela Medical, or 140 milliseconds in Medtronic devices. Some devices allow the patient to tag a time point when they have symptoms, or even store an electrogram in the ICD at such a moment. In some athletic patients these event recorder functions of devices can be used to check for possible electromagnetic interference in their specific athletic surroundings, or detection or exclusion of arrhythmias at the time of symptoms.

Over recent years, technology has emerged that allows wireless transfer of measured parameters and of shock-related information to central servers, from where physicians can be alerted (SMS, fax, internet) and via which they can review device function and recorded episodes. In the near future, most devices will also perform automatic ventricular or atrial capture monitoring, which will complete the pallet of remotely monitored parameters. These remote monitoring systems may allow earlier detection of situations that could potentially lead to inappropriate shocks (such as atrial arrhythmias or lead insulation defects) and could therefore improve quality of life in young ICD patients.

Therapy of inappropriate shocks is mainly preventing them

One should be critical of the R and T wave amplitude, morphology, and ratio during implant, to ensure correct sensing without T wave oversensing. The atrial electrogram should also be evaluated on the absence of far-field R-wave sensing. ICD technology is developed to detect small electrograms during ventricular fibrillation. Because the ventricular lead is implanted in the RV, which in some athletes may be diseased, the recorded electrograms may be of small amplitude and prone to undersensing of VF or delayed shock delivery, which is also is a risky complication [40]. This stresses the importance for optimal positioning of the leads during the implantation procedure so that they have correct sensing, ensuring reliable VF detection and minimizing the risk for double counting and inappropriate shocks.

Rational selection of device and leads and the programming of rate zones and related therapies have been discussed above. Moreover, Fig. 1 illustrates that atrial information does rarely prevent shock delivery if the VT- or VF-zone rate limits have been exceeded. If any supraventricular arrhythmia that can be ablated is known in the patient, it is worthwhile to consider prophylactic ablation to prevent rapid atrio-ventricular conduction during later physical activity, which could result in inappropriate shocks. Physically active patients should be counseled on the possibility of electromagnetic interference, and occurrences of such interference excluded during follow-up visits.

The most important preventive action in athletic people is to anticipate and prevent sinus tachycardia. An exercise test or long-term ambulatory ECG recording during the sports activities of the patient may provide very valuable information in this regard. Inappropriate therapy, caused by sinus tachycardia, can be prevented by limiting the amount of maximal exercise, warning against sudden bursts of exercise, and prophylactic administration of AV nodal slowing drugs (like beta-blockers, or calcium antagonists, or digoxin). This applies not only to the fittest patients, but also to patients with a history of atrial arrhythmias or patients with heart failure (who have a higher risk for development of atrial fibrillation).

Before elective surgery, it is recommended to temporarily program off tachyarrhythmia detection and therapy, although interference with the radiofrequency currents emitted by electrosurgical units is very rare in modern devices. Although a magnet can be applied for temporary inhibition, it may slide off during the intervention or even may be forgotten to be taken away after the intervention. Programmer based inactivation and

A

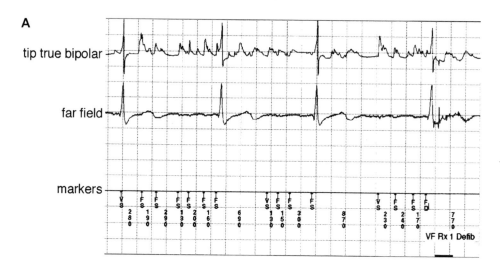

tip true bipolar

far field

markers

B

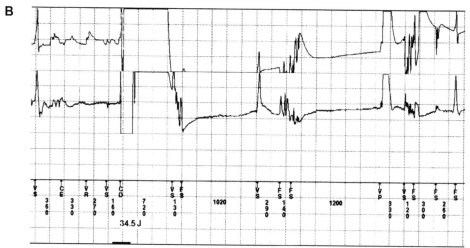

C

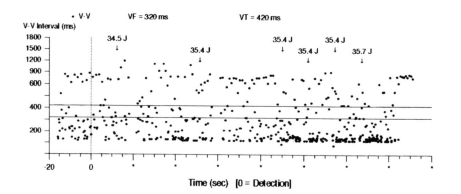

ID#	Date/Time	Type	V. Cycle	Last Rx	Success	Duration
4	May 08 11:28:12	VF	370 ms	VF Rx 6	No	7.5 min

reactivation is therefore preferred; after the surgical intervention, this also allows a system check and integrity check of the leads.

Preventing other inappropriate shocks can be challenging, with different treatment options available to the electrophysiologist: reprogramming, drug treatment, ablation, further restriction of activity, often in combination. In some patients, repositioning or replacement of the lead may be required. Lead extraction is feasible in a majority of patients but is not without risk [41]. Therefore, if fewer leads were inserted at the initial implantation, the higher the chance that one can opt to implant an additional lead, a policy which in young people can prevent risky extraction procedures early in life. In some patients with inappropriate shocks, upgrading from a VVI-device to DDD-device can be considered to prevent further inappropriate shocks, although this requires a careful evaluation whether the atrial electrogram information would really allow a better discrimination by the device.

Last but not least, patients who experience inappropriate shocks need psychologic support and often supporting therapy. It takes time and guidance to reassure them again of an active life style, with carefully titrated physical activities. A systematic psychologic support team may be helpful, but is not everywhere available. At minimum, elaborate counseling and reassuring by the treating physician or electrophysiologist is needed. Even then, it may take months before the patient resumes a normal life-style and dares to perform any new physical activities. It has been reported that participation of ICD patients in systematic rehabilitation programs, including psychologic counseling, leads to better reintegration and psychologic well being [18,42]. An international trial (Relax-ICD) is underway to evaluate this in larger ICD patients groups, although this

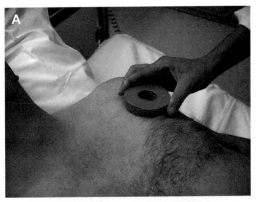

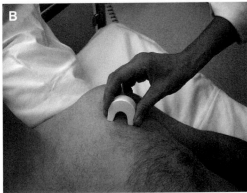

Fig. 7. Inhibition of tachyarrhythmia therapy (antitachypacing or shocks) by magnet application. It is recommended to use a stronger doughnut shaped magnet (A), but also regular pacemaker magnets (like the one shown in (B) can inhibit ICD therapy delivery. In older models, application for more than 30 seconds could permanently turn off the device, but this is almost never the case today. Nevertheless, it is recommended to verify the magnet behavior of the implanted ICD (see Table 1) and to interrogate the ICD with a programmer to evaluate its functional status. Except for Sorin/Ela Medical devices, bradycardia function is not affected, and is never inhibited.

Fig. 6. Insulation defect leading to repetitive inappropriate shocks. (A) During sinus bradycardia of 45/min, the sensing bipole channel in this athlete with an ICD recorded spurious electrograms with a high rate, which were detected by the ICD within the VF zone and led to inappropriate detection. The patient was sitting at that time. The electrograms were the result of abrasion of the insulator of the pacing/sensing conductors, while the far-field electrogram (recorded between the shock coil in the RV and the ICD can) initially showed normal tracings. (B) After the first shock (35 J), the artifacts increased in magnitude and now were also present on the far-field electrograms. (C) Interval plot showing the very wide scatter on the recorded R-R intervals, with much more variation than seen during atrial fibrillation and especially with very short intervals. After the 6th shock, the device stopped therapy delivery, despite continuation of the artifacts. Later however, intermittent episodes without artifacts (see right side) led to "arrhythmia termination" classification by the device, resulting in a new six-shock inappropriate therapy sequence within a few minutes. When the patient entered the hospital, he had received more than 25 shocks and was frightened.

Table 1
Magnet behavior of ICDs

	Biotronik	Guidant (Boston Scientific)	Medtronic	Sorin (Ela-Medical)	St. Jude
Inhibition tachy detection?	yes	no if "monitoring only" (except electro-cautery mode)	yes	yes	yes
Inhibition tachy therapy?	yes	yes	yes	yes	yes
Permanent deactivation?	no	yes until 1999	no	no	no
Different old versus new?	no	yes (ICDs < Prizm 1999)	no	no	no
Programmable?	no	yes if :1) "OFF after 30 sec" (devices until Aug 2004) 2) "no effect" (also if "Pt monitor On")	no	no	yes if "no effect"
Effect on Brady behavior?	no	no (except "electrocautery mode": VOO or DOO)	no	magnet rate function of battery voltage, in programmed mode (max output; ≤96/') (Defender <1995: DOO or VOO)	no
Interrogation possible?	yes (obligatory)	yes	yes (obligatory)	no	no

study does not specifically address a young and athletic patient population.

Summary

Implantable defibrillators provide a very important tool to prevent sudden arrhythmic death in athletes, or physically active people with an inherited risk for malignant ventricular arrhythmias. They often provide a means for safe continuation of mild to moderate recreational sports activity.

Long-term acceptance of the therapy and quality of life will be highly dependent on the prevention of inappropriate therapy. As this text has outlined, prevention requires serious anticipation from physician and patient. A choice for as few and as simple leads as possible ensuring durable functioning, devices with high longevity, careful programming tailored to the characteristics of the patient's physiologic and pathologic heart rhythms, preventive bradycardic medication, and rehabilitation with psychologic counseling, are all very important in this respect. Nevertheless, the patient or athlete also has to accept some limitations, such as restricting the intensity of sports participation and accepting the intake of prophylactic bradycardic agents. However, with these concerted measures, the sword of Damocles' threat of imminent sudden death or inappropriate shocks can largely be removed, allowing continuation of an active young life in most.

References

[1] Zipes DP, Camm AJ, Borggrefe M, et al. ACC/AHA/ESC 2006 guidelines for management of patients with ventricular arrhythmias and the prevention of sudden cardiac death—executive summary: a report of the American College of Cardiology/American Heart Association Task Force and the European Society of Cardiology Committee for Practice Guidelines (Writing Committee to Develop Guidelines for Management of Patients with Ventricular Arrhythmias and the Prevention of Sudden Cardiac Death) Developed in collaboration with the European Heart Rhythm Association and the Heart Rhythm Society. Eur Heart J 2006;27(17):2099–140.

[2] Zipes DP, Ackerman MJ, Estes NA 3rd, et al. 36th Bethesda Conference: eligibility recommendations for competitive athletes with cardiovascular abnormalities-general considerations. Task Force 7: arrhythmias. J Am Coll Cardiol 2005;45(8): 1354–63.

[3] Maron BJ, Chaitman BR, Ackerman MJ, et al. Recommendations for physical activity and recreational sports participation for young patients with genetic cardiovascular diseases. Circulation 2004;109(22): 2807–16.

[4] Pelliccia A, Fagard R, Bjornstad HH, et al. Recommendations for competitive sports participation in athletes with cardiovascular disease: a consensus document from the Study Group of Sports Cardiology of the Working Group of Cardiac Rehabilitation and Exercise Physiology and the Working Group of Myocardial and Pericardial Diseases of the European Society of Cardiology. Eur Heart J 2005;26(14):1422–45.

[5] Heidbuchel H, Corrado D, Biffi A, et al. Recommendations for participation in leisure-time physical activity and competitive sports of patients with arrhythmias and potentially arrhythmogenic conditions, part II: ventricular arrhythmias, channelopathies and implantable defibrillators. Eur J Cardiovasc Prev Rehabil 2006;13(5):676–86.

[6] Corrado D, Pelliccia A, Bjornstad HH, et al. Cardiovascular pre-participation screening of young competitive athletes for prevention of sudden death: proposal for a common European protocol. Consensus Statement of the Study Group of Sport Cardiology of the Working Group of Cardiac Rehabilitation and Exercise Physiology and the Working Group of Myocardial and Pericardial Diseases of the European Society of Cardiology. Eur Heart J 2005; 26(5):516–24.

[7] Wathen MS, DeGroot PJ, Sweeney MO, et al. Prospective randomized multicenter trial of empirical antitachycardia pacing versus shocks for spontaneous rapid ventricular tachycardia in patients with implantable cardioverter-defibrillators: pacing fast ventricular tachycardia reduces shock therapies (PainFREE Rx II) trial results. Circulation 2004; 110(17):2591–6.

[8] Deisenhofer I, Kolb C, Ndrepepa G, et al. Do current dual chamber cardioverter defibrillators have advantages over conventional single chamber cardioverter defibrillators in reducing inappropriate therapies? A randomized, prospective study. J Cardiovasc Electrophysiol 2001;12(2):134–42.

[9] Sinha AM, Stellbrink C, Schuchert A, et al. Clinical experience with a new detection algorithm for differentiation of supraventricular from ventricular tachycardia in a dual-chamber defibrillator. J Cardiovasc Electrophysiol 2004;15(6):646–52.

[10] Berger RD, Lerew DR, Smith JM, et al. The Rhythm ID Going Head to Head Trial (RIGHT): design of a randomized trial comparing competitive rhythm discrimination algorithms in implantable cardioverter defibrillators. J Cardiovasc Electrophysiol 2006;17(7):749–53.

[11] Connolly SJ, Kerr CR, Gent M, et al. Effects of physiologic pacing versus ventricular pacing on the risk of stroke and death due to cardiovascular causes. Canadian Trial of Physiologic Pacing Investigators. N Engl J Med 2000;342(19):1385–91.

[12] Ellenbogen KA, Wood MA, Shepard RK, et al. Detection and management of an implantable cardioverter defibrillator lead failure: incidence and clinical implications. J Am Coll Cardiol 2003;41(1): 73–80.

[13] Dorwarth U, Frey B, Dugas M, et al. Transvenous defibrillation leads: high incidence of failure during long-term follow-up. J Cardiovasc Electrophysiol 2003;14(1):38–43.

[14] Lamas GA, Keefe JM. The effects of equitation (horseback riding) on a motion responsive DDDR pacemaker. Pacing Clin Electrophysiol 1990;13(11 Pt 1):1371–3.

[15] Alt E, Combs W, Willhaus R, et al. A comparative study of activity and dual sensor: activity and minute ventilation pacing responses to ascending and descending stairs. Pacing Clin Electrophysiol 1998; 21(10):1862–8.

[16] Maron BJ, Mitten MJ, Quandt EF, et al. Competitive athletes with cardiovascular disease—the case of Nicholas Knapp. N Engl J Med 1998;339(22): 1632–5.

[17] Mitchell JH, Haskell W, Snell P, et al. Task Force 8: classification of sports. J Am Coll Cardiol 2005; 45(8):1364–7.

[18] Vanhees L, Kornaat M, Defoor J, et al. Effect of exercise training in patients with an implantable cardioverter defibrillator. Eur Heart J 2004;25(13): 1120–6.

[19] Lampert R, Cannom D, Olshansky B. Safety of sports participation in patients with implantable cardioverter defibrillators: a survey of heart rhythm society members. J Cardiovasc Electrophysiol 2006; 17(1):11–5.

[20] Sakakibara Y. Delayed pinpoint exposure of a pacemaker following seat belt trauma. Pacing Clin Electrophysiol 1997;20(2 Pt 1):370–1.

[21] Schuger CD, Mittleman R, Habbal B, et al. Ventricular lead transection and atrial lead damage in a young softball player shortly after the insertion of a permanent pacemaker. Pacing Clin Electrophysiol 1992;15(9):1236–9.

[22] Deering JA, Pederson DN. A case of pacemaker lead fracture associated with weightlifting. Pacing Clin Electrophysiol 1992;15(9):1354–5.

[23] Gould L, Betzu R, Taddeo M, et al. Pulse generator failure due to blunt trauma. Clin Cardiol 1988;11(8): 581–2.

[24] Grieco JG, Scanlon PJ, Pifarre R. Pacing lead fracture after a deceleration injury. Ann Thorac Surg 1989;47(3):453–4.

[25] Pinski SL, Fahy GJ. The proarrhythmic potential of implantable cardioverter-defibrillators. Circulation 1995;92(6):1651–64.

[26] Rosenqvist M, Beyer T, Block M, et al. Adverse events with transvenous implantable cardioverter-defibrillators: a prospective multicenter study. European 7219 Jewel ICD investigators. Circulation 1998;98(7):663–70.

[27] Gradaus R, Block M, Brachmann J, et al. Mortality, morbidity, and complications in 3344 patients with implantable cardioverter defibrillators: results from the German ICD Registry EURID. Pacing Clin Electrophysiol 2003;26(7 Pt 1):1511–8.

[28] Nanthakumar K, Dorian P, Paquette M, et al. Is inappropriate implantable defibrillator shock therapy predictable? J Interv Card Electrophysiol 2003; 8(3):215–20.

[29] Weretka S, Michaelsen J, Becker R, et al. Ventricular oversensing: a study of 101 patients implanted with dual chamber defibrillators and two different lead systems. Pacing Clin Electrophysiol 2003; 26(1 Pt 1):65–70.

[30] Healy E, Ngarmukos T, Rosenthal L. A case of bad timing: inappropriate implantable cardioverter defibrillator therapy due to a critically placed premature ventricular contraction. Pacing Clin Electrophysiol 2002;25(9):1403–5.

[31] Schimpf R, Wolpert C, Bianchi F, et al. Congenital short QT syndrome and implantable cardioverter defibrillator treatment: inherent risk for inappropriate shock delivery. J Cardiovasc Electrophysiol 2003;14(12):1273–7.

[32] Vijayaraman P, Ferrell MS, Rhee B, et al. Implantable cardioverter defibrillator oversensing: what is the mechanism? J Cardiovasc Electrophysiol 2004; 15(6):723–4.

[33] Casavant D, Haffajee C, Stevens S, et al. Aborted implantable cardioverter defibrillator shock during facial electrosurgery. Pacing Clin Electrophysiol 1998;21(6):1325–6.

[34] Garg A, Wadhwa M, Brown K, et al. Inappropriate implantable cardioverter defibrillator discharge from sensing of external alternating current leak. J Interv Card Electrophysiol 2002; 7(2):181–4.

[35] Vlay SC. Fish pond electromagnetic interference resulting in an inappropriate implantable cardioverter defibrillator shock. Pacing Clin Electrophysiol 2002;25(10):1532.

[36] Kolb C, Schmieder S, Schmitt C. Inappropriate shock delivery due to interference between a washing machine and an implantable cardioverter defibrillator. J Interv Card Electrophysiol 2002;7(3): 255–6.

[37] Anfinsen OG, Berntsen RF, Aass H, et al. Implantable cardioverter defibrillator dysfunction during and after magnetic resonance imaging. Pacing Clin Electrophysiol 2002;25(9):1400–2.

[38] Mewis C, Kuhlkamp V, Dornberger V, et al. High incidence of isolator fractures in transvenous implantation of cardioverter defibrillators [German]. Z Kardiol 1997;86(2):85–94.

[39] De Lurgio DB, Sathavorn C, Mera F, et al. Incidence and implications of abrasion of implantable cardioverter-defibrillator leads. Am J Cardiol 1997; 79(10):1409–11.

[40] Dekker LR, Schrama TA, Steinmetz FH, et al. Undersensing of VF in a patient with optimal R wave sensing during sinus rhythm. Pacing Clin Electrophysiol 2004;27(6 Pt 1):833–4.

[41] Bracke F, Meijer A, Van Gelder B. Extraction of pacemaker and implantable cardioverter defibrillator leads: patient and lead characteristics in relation to the requirement of extraction tools. Pacing Clin Electrophysiol 2002;25(7):1037–40.

[42] Fitchet A, Doherty PJ, Bundy C, et al. Comprehensive cardiac rehabilitation programme for implantable cardioverter-defibrillator patients: a randomised controlled trial. Heart 2003;89(2): 155–60.

Index

Note: Page numbers of article titles are in **boldface** type.

United States Postal Service

Statement of Ownership, Management, and Circulation
(All Periodicals Publications Except Requestor Publications)

1. Publication Title
Cardiology Clinics

2. Publication Number
0 0 0 - 7 0 1

3. Filing Date
9/14/07

4. Issue Frequency
Feb, May, Aug, Nov

5. Number of Issues Published Annually
4

6. Annual Subscription Price
$198.00

7. Complete Mailing Address of Known Office of Publication (Not printer) (Street, city, county, state, and ZIP+4)

Elsevier Inc.
360 Park Avenue South
New York, NY 10010-1710

Contact Person
Stephen Bushing

Telephone (Include area code)
215-239-3688

8. Complete Mailing Address of Headquarters or General Business Office of Publisher (Not printer)

Elsevier Inc., 360 Park Avenue South, New York, NY 10010-1710

9. Full Names and Complete Mailing Addresses of Publisher, Editor, and Managing Editor (Do not leave blank)

Publisher (Name and complete mailing address)

John Schrefer, Elsevier, Inc., 1600 John F. Kennedy Blvd. Suite 1800, Philadelphia, PA 19103-2899

Editor (Name and complete mailing address)

Barbara Cohen-Kligerman, Elsevier, Inc., 1600 John F. Kennedy Blvd. Suite 1800, Philadelphia, PA 19103-2899

Managing Editor (Name and complete mailing address)

Catherine Bewick, Elsevier, Inc., 1600 John F. Kennedy Blvd. Suite 1800, Philadelphia, PA 19103-2899

10. Owner (Do not leave blank. If the publication is owned by a corporation, give the name and address of the corporation immediately followed by the names and addresses of all stockholders owning or holding 1 percent or more of the total amount of stock. If not owned by a corporation, give the names and addresses of the individual owners. If owned by a partnership or other unincorporated firm, give its name and address as well as those of each individual owner. If the publication is published by a nonprofit organization, give its name and address.)

Full Name	Complete Mailing Address
Wholly owned subsidiary of	4520 East-West Highway
Reed/Elsevier, US holdings	Bethesda, MD 20814

11. Known Bondholders, Mortgagees, and Other Security Holders Owning or Holding 1 Percent or More of Total Amount of Bonds, Mortgages, or Other Securities. If none, check box ☐ None

Full Name	Complete Mailing Address
N/A	

12. Tax Status (For completion by nonprofit organizations authorized to mail at nonprofit rates) (Check one)
The purpose, function, and nonprofit status of this organization and the exempt status for federal income tax purposes:
☐ Has Not Changed During Preceding 12 Months
☐ Has Changed During Preceding 12 Months (Publisher must submit explanation of change with this statement)

PS Form 3526, September 2006 (Page 1 of 3) (Instructions Page 3) PSN 7530-01-000-9931 **PRIVACY NOTICE**: See our Privacy policy in www.usps.com

---

13. Publication Title
Cardiology Clinics of North America

14. Issue Date for Circulation Data Below
May 2007

15. Extent and Nature of Circulation

		Average No. Copies Each Issue During Preceding 12 Months	No. Copies of Single Issue Published Nearest to Filing Date
a. Total Number of Copies (Net press run)		2575	2500
b. Paid Circulation (By Mail and Outside the Mail)	(1) Mailed Outside-County Paid Subscriptions Stated on PS Form 3541 (Include paid distribution above nominal rate, advertiser's proof copies, and exchange copies)	1174	1085
	(2) Mailed In-County Paid Subscriptions Stated on PS Form 3541 (Include paid distribution above nominal rate, advertiser's proof copies, and exchange copies)		
	(3) Paid Distribution Outside the Mails Including Sales Through Dealers and Carriers, Street Vendors, Counter Sales, and Other Paid Distribution Outside USPS®	570	516
	(4) Paid Distribution by Other Classes Mailed Through the USPS (e.g. First-Class Mail®)		
c. Total Paid Distribution (Sum of 15b (1), (2), (3), and (4))	▶	1744	1601
d. Free or Nominal Rate Distribution (By Mail and Outside the Mail)	(1) Free or Nominal Rate Outside-County Copies Included on PS Form 3541	100	60
	(2) Free or Nominal Rate In-County Copies Included on PS Form 3541		
	(3) Free or Nominal Rate Copies Mailed at Other Classes Mailed Through the USPS (e.g. First-Class Mail)		
	(4) Free or Nominal Rate Distribution Outside the Mail (Carriers or other means)		
e. Total Free or Nominal Rate Distribution (Sum of 15d (1), (2), (3) and (4))	▶	100	60
f. Total Distribution (Sum of 15c and 15e)	▶	1844	1661
g. Copies not Distributed (See instructions to publishers #4 (page #3))	▶	731	839
h. Total (Sum of 15f and g)	▶	2575	2500
i. Percent Paid (15c divided by 15f times 100)		94.58%	96.39%

16. Publication of Statement of Ownership
If the publication is a general publication, publication of this statement is required. Will be printed ☐ Publication not required
in the November 2007 issue of this publication.

17. Signature and Title of Editor, Publisher, Business Manager, or Owner

[signature]

Date September 14, 2007

Bob Fanucci – Executive Director of Subscription Services

I certify that all information furnished on this form is true and complete. I understand that anyone who furnishes false or misleading information on this form or who omits material or information requested on the form may be subject to criminal sanctions (including fines and imprisonment) and/or civil sanctions (including civil penalties)

PS Form 3526, September 2006 (Page 2 of 3)

Moving?

Make sure your subscription moves with you!

To notify us of your new address, find your **Clinics Account Number** (located on your mailing label above your name), and contact customer service at:

E-mail: elspcs@elsevier.com

800-654-2452 (subscribers in the U.S. & Canada)
407-345-4000 (subscribers outside of the U.S. & Canada)

Fax number: 407-363-9661

Elsevier Periodicals Customer Service
6277 Sea Harbor Drive
Orlando, FL 32887-4800

*To ensure uninterrupted delivery of your subscription, please notify us at least 4 weeks in advance of move.

ELSEVIER